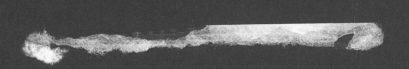

SLIMMING WORLD's
30-minute
meals

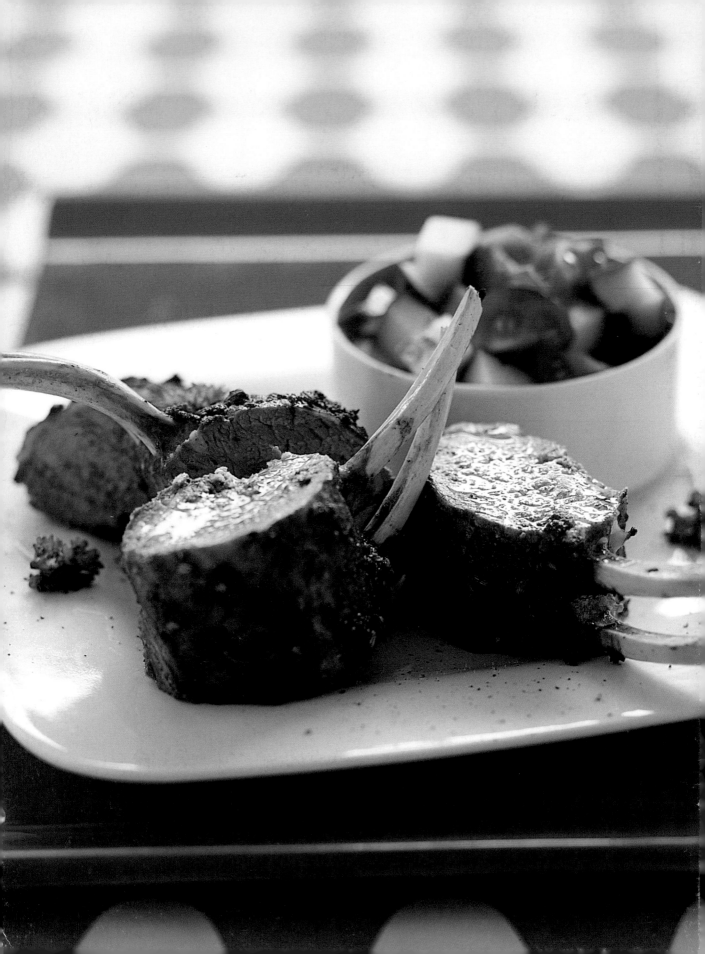

SLIMMING WORLD's
30-minute
meals

120 quick recipes for family feasts

EBURY
PRESS

First published in 2007
10 9 8 7 6 5 4 3 2 1

Ebury Publishing
Random House, 20 Vauxhall Bridge Road, London SW1V 2SA

Random House Australia (Pty) Limited
20 Alfred Street, Milsons Point, Sydney, New South Wales 2061, Australia

Random House New Zealand Limited
18 Poland Road, Glenfield, Auckland 10, New Zealand

Random House South Africa (Pty) Limited
Isle of Houghton, Corner Boundary Road & Carse O'Gowrie, Houghton, 2198, South Africa

Random House Publishers India Private Limited
301 World Trade Tower, Hotel Intercontinental Grand Complex, Barakhamba Lane, New Delhi 110 001, India

The Random House Group Limited Reg. No. 954009
www.randomhouse.co.uk

A CIP catalogue record for this book is available from the British Library.

ISBN-13: 9780091914332

Recipes created by Sunil Vijayakar
Editor: Emma Callery
Design: Nicky Barneby

Food photography: Jon Whitaker
Food stylist: Sunil Vijayakar
Prop stylist: Rachel Jukes

For Slimming World
Founder and Chairman: Margaret Miles-Bramwell
Managing Director: Caryl Richards
Project co-ordinators: Allison Brentnall and Beverley Farnsworth
Text by Sheila Ashton

Papers used by Ebury Press are natural, recyclable products made from wood grown in sustainable forests.

Printed and bound in China by C&C Offset Printing Co. Ltd

cookery
notes

- Both metric and imperial measures are given for the recipes. Follow either set of measures as they are not interchangeable.
- All spoon measures are level: 1 tsp = 5ml spoon, 1 tbsp = 15ml spoon.
- ⓥ Suitable for vegetarians
- ❋ Suitable for freezing
- Ovens should be preheated to the specified temperature. Grills should also be preheated.
- Use large eggs unless otherwise specified.
- Note that some of the recipes contain lightly cooked eggs. Avoid serving these to anyone who is pregnant or in a vulnerable health group, because of the small risk of salmonella infection.
- Always use fresh herbs, unless dried herbs are suggested in the recipe.
- Use freshly ground black pepper and sea salt unless otherwise specified.

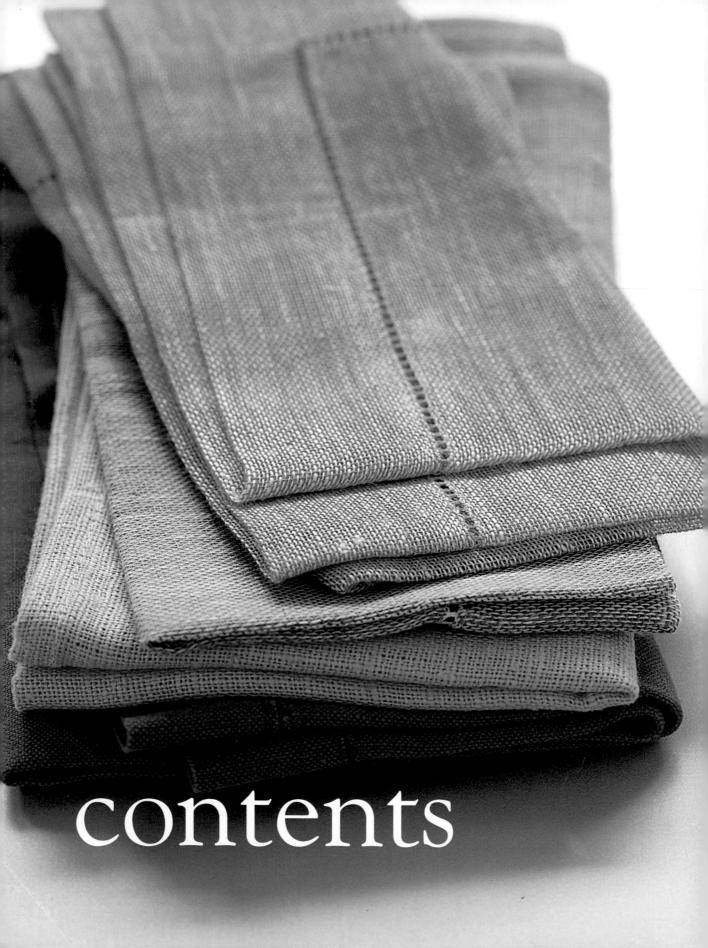

contents

foreword

Dear Food Lover,

Welcome to the newest, temptingly mouth-watering addition to Slimming World's family of recipe books. With bookshop shelves groaning under the weight of so many sumptuous-looking titles, it's great you know you can trust us to satisfy your family's needs and fit in with your busy lifestyle. Rest assured, this book won't disappoint.

Bring back the happy times when families came together for their main meal of the day. If you want ways to please a hungry household without compromising on health; if you want to lose weight without feeling deprived; if you want to save time and money without skimping on quality; if you simply want to get back round the dining table together, *Slimming World's 30-Minute Meals* are for you!

The pages that follow are packed to the brim with delicious dishes that you can whip up in just half an hour and enjoy together at leisure. Each has been carefully developed with both weight control and the needs of the family in mind and follows the very latest nutrition guidelines. Isn't it good to know that, with all the demands placed on us in this fast-paced, modern world, where family weight and health issues have never been more acute, we can all be free to enjoy our food – and family life – to the full?

Food Optimising© is the eating plan that lies at the very heart of Slimming World. Freedom is the key. All the recipes in this book, using ordinary, everyday foods, are Food Optimising meals with 'Free Food'® as their base. Prepare to be amazed that you can have all this taste and all this food and still lose weight. Food Optimising has been Slimming World's cornerstone ever since its inception 37 years ago – with dramatic success! As well as bringing this amazing weight-loss system to the rescue of slimmers everywhere, my passionate desire was then – and remains to this day – the development of a support system that recognises what spurs us on or holds us back from living our dreams and that is actually effective in bringing those dreams to reality.

At Slimming World we're driven by a fervent belief that every one of us deserves to be free – free from guilt, free to set our own goals, free to enjoy our food, free to live life to the full and, most importantly, free to be ourselves. That's why, in a Slimming World group, no one is ever judged, preached to, humiliated or pressurised on their journey to their personal target. You plan your own route. We're just shining a light on your personal map to success.

That same conviction drives our most recent pioneering initiative, Family Affair. In an age when the problem of obesity – among children and young people as well as adults – continues to climb alarmingly, we know that the real long-term answers lie within the home, within the family. That's why we've taken a bold, family-based approach to healthy eating that empowers families to change their lifestyle jointly. Attending a Slimming World group together, families can not only enjoy the expertise, understanding and support of their Consultant and fellow group members, they can reinforce their new approach to a healthier lifestyle by planning meals and creating dishes together and motivating each other at home. Generous, versatile and nutritionally balanced, Food Optimising has also been made even more liberal to meet the needs of young people, with whom our focus is on health and vitality, rather than on weight.

So please use this book to the full. You'll find these fabulously tasty menus will allow you the freedom to make family mealtimes an all-round guilt-free pleasure. And if you're looking for support to overcome your own or your family's weight issues, remember, we're here, ready to welcome you into the Slimming World family. The door to success is always open at Slimming World and you'll find the friendliest of welcomes.

With warmest wishes,

Margaret Miles-Bramwell
Founder and Chairman

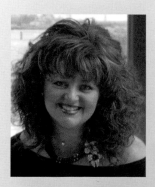

fast feasting!

Your family's health and happiness matters to you, that's plain from the fact you've picked up this book! It's also clear you love food. So how can you stay in control when, as a nation, we know more about health and nutrition than any previous generation, yet we've never been heavier, more unhealthy or more pushed for time?

Perhaps you have concerns about your own weight or the weight of other family members. Maybe you want to curb excess calories but don't have time for tiresome counting. Or are you simply looking for delicious family meals that leave you satisfied rather than guilty – and don't need hours of preparation?

Whatever led you our way, you will find this book stuffed to the brim with deliciously satisfying dishes designed to tantalise your taste buds without expanding your waistline. Each inspirationally delectable meal has been created by Sunil Vijayakar, the mastermind behind thousands of Slimming World recipes, with three things in mind – the marriage of healthy eating, fantastic flavours and oh-so-easy preparation.

FOOD OPTIMISING

Every one of Sunil's mouth-watering recipes is based on the most generous, effective and flexible weight-loss system there is. Food Optimising, the ingeniously simple system at the heart of the Slimming World phenomenon, is quite simply a healthy life plan for food lovers.

It's nothing to do with fads and everything to do with choice. It was developed by Slimming World chairman and founder, Margaret Miles-Bramwell, nearly 40 years ago, borne out of her personal struggle with weight. Based on a scientific understanding of the satisfaction of appetite, the psychology of slimming and the latest nutrition guidelines, Food Optimising gives slimmers the power to enjoy 'real' food – from steak, pasta and potatoes to chips and chocolate – and still lose weight beautifully. Crucially, the choice is always in their hands.

In fact, Food Optimising is all about choice. It features five daily menu options, Green, Original, Mix2Max, Success Express and Free2Go, which provide limitless choices for all ages, tastes and lifestyles. The mainstay of each is a massive list of Free Foods – nutrient-rich foods that satisfy the appetite without packing calories, leaving you feeling fuller for longer. You are free to enjoy these without limit. Original-day Free Foods include lean meat, bacon, poultry, fish and seafood while Green-day Free Foods include rice, pasta, beans and potatoes.

In addition to mountains of Free Foods, Food Optimising offers measured portions of foods that add fibre, vitamins and minerals – especially calcium. As all are important to your health, we call them Healthy Extras. And still there is more – extra treats that bring added pleasure to our daily menus. We refer to these as 'Syns' (short for synergy), and you can discover more about them and about Food Optimising on page 202.

FAMILY AFFAIR

Food Optimising gives you the freedom to throw away calorie counters and 'banned' food lists, freedom to eat out, freedom to pile the plate high and still lose weight and be healthy. That's a high priority for any parent keen to ensure the long-term health of their children. Recognising this led Slimming World to become the first national organisation in the UK to address the worrying issue of weight and the younger generation through Family Affair, a scheme that opens the doors to a healthier lifestyle for whole families who can mutually benefit from our expertise, warmth and support. And the latest innovation welcomes children aged from 11 to 15. Find out more on page 209.

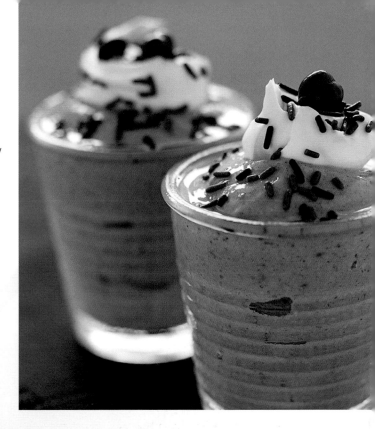

IMAGE THERAPY

All too often the heaviest burden a slimmer has to bear is not temptation or lack of knowledge but rather the feelings of guilt, failure and despair that can sink a slimming plan. No one understands this better than Slimming World. The warm, friendly upbeat atmosphere of Slimming World group meetings is no accident. It is built deliberately out of a conviction that long-term weight management is not about 'just eating less' or 'calories-in versus calories-out'. It's about valuing self-esteem and self-worth; it's about sharing and support. At a Slimming World meeting, highly trained Consultants encourage the group to take part in a unique system of problem-solving, motivation and inspiration – Image Therapy – explained on page 205.

BODY MAGIC

Healthy eating brings enormous benefits to our sense of well-being and this can be boosted by becoming more active – and no, that doesn't have to involve gruelling workouts at the gym. Regular, moderate activity – such as walking the dog, getting off the bus a stop early, walking to school instead of driving – can bring tremendous benefits. And that's why everyone is encouraged to make it part of the Slimming World experience.

Rather than 'prescribing' activities for its members, Slimming World puts the choice in their hands. Body Magic is a programme that recognises and rewards members for small increases in activity levels and encourages them to make it part of their everyday routine (see page 207).

If you are looking for some great-tasting meal ideas, feel free to read on. If you want the time to make mealtimes a family experience, feel free to eat and enjoy. And if you are concerned about your weight or that of someone you love, then please ... feel free to browse or get the most out of everything this book has to offer.

syn-free
storecupboard

All these storecupboard ingredients are Free Foods for both Green and Original days, unless otherwise stated.

CANS AND BOTTLES
Artificial sweetener
Baked beans in tomato sauce (Green days only)
Borlotti beans (Green days only)
Butter beans (Green days only)
Cannellini beans (Green days only)
Capers
Chickpeas (Green days only)
Red kidney beans (Green days only)

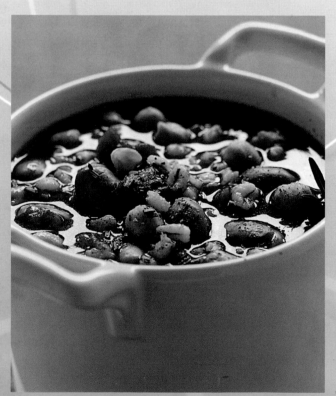

Lean canned ham (Original days only)
Mixed beans (Green days only)
Sweetcorn (Green days only)
Tomatoes, plum and chopped

FROM THE FRIDGE
Chillies, red and green
Fresh herbs, e.g.
  basil
  bay leaf
  chives
  coriander
  dill
  kaffir lime leaves
  lemongrass
  mint
  oregano
  parsley (standard and flat-leaf)
  rosemary
  tarragon
  thyme
Ginger, fresh root
Quark soft cheese
Very low fat natural cottage cheese
Very low fat natural fromage frais
Very low fat natural yogurt

STAPLES
Barley (Green days only)
Bovril stock: all varieties
Bulgur wheat (Green days only)

Couscous (Green days only)

Dried red chilli flakes

Fat-free dressings, French-style and vinaigrette

Fry Light

Garlic granules

Herbs and ground and whole spices, e.g.

    bouquet garni (thyme, bay leaves and parsley)

    Cajun spice

    cardamom seeds

    cayenne pepper

    chilli powder (mild, medium and hot)

    Chinese five-spice

    cinnamon (ground and sticks)

    coriander (ground and seeds)

    cumin (ground and seeds)

    curry powder (mild to hot)

    dried bay leaves

    dried mint

    fennel seeds

    ground ginger

    mixed dried herbs: all varieties

    mustard seeds (black)

    nutmeg

    oregano

    paprika (mild and sweet smoked)

    pimenton

    pink and mixed peppercorns

    saffron threads

    tandoori spice powder

Lentils, all varieties (Green days only)

Mustard powder

Passata (sieved tomatoes)

Quinoa (Green days only)

Pasta and noodles, all types, dried
    (Green days only)

Rice noodles (Green days only)

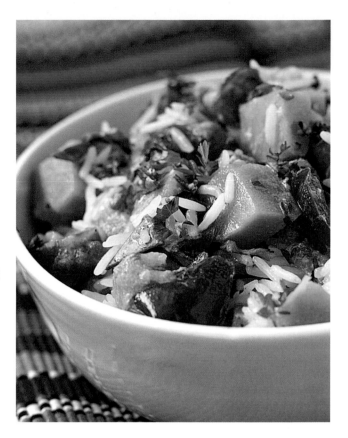

Rice: all varieties (Green days only), e.g.

    Arborio

    basmati

    brown

    long grain

    risotto

    wild

Sea salt

Soy sauces, dark and light

Tabasco sauce

Vanilla essence/extract

Vecon

Vinegars: e.g. balsamic, raspberry, red wine

Worcestershire sauce

ON THE KITCHEN WORKTOP

Eggs

Garlic

Lemons and limes

Onions and shallots

Tomatoes, all kinds

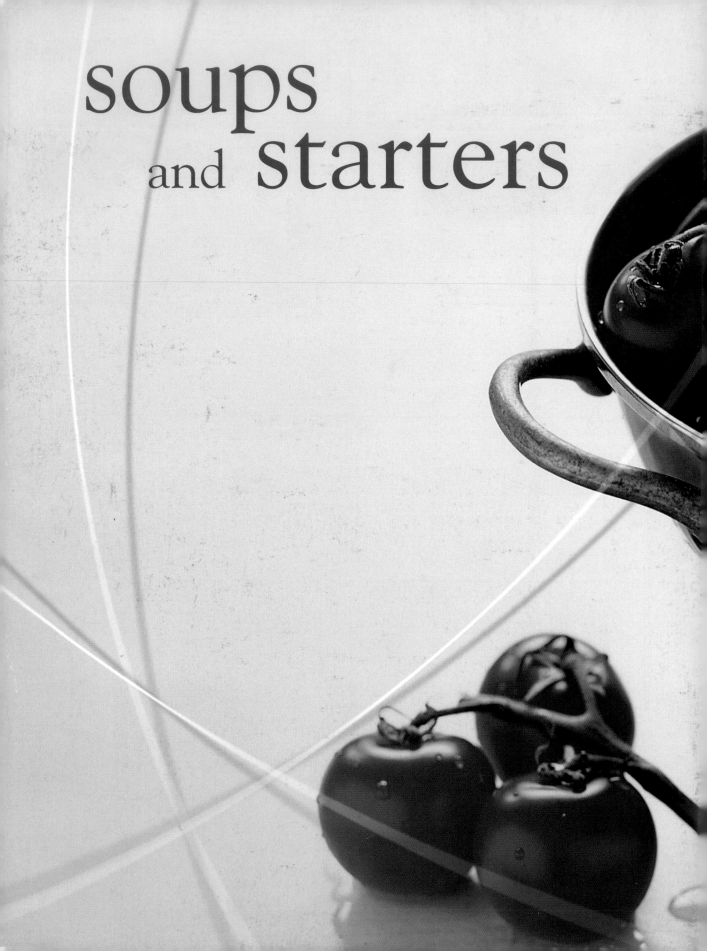

soups
and starters

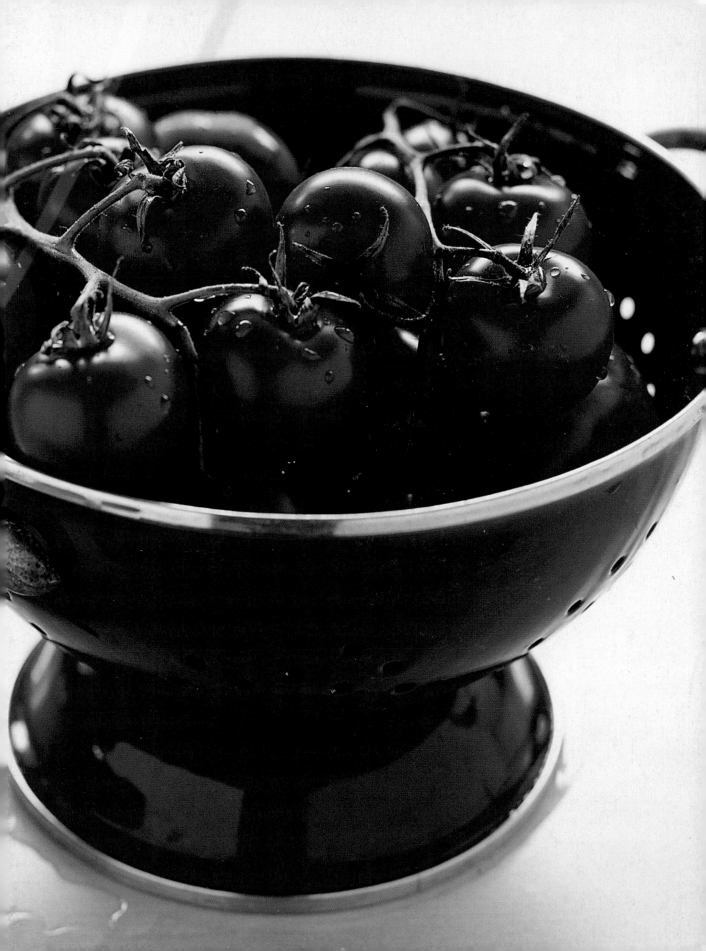

tomato, rice
and pea soup

Prepared in minutes, this colourful and hearty twist to tomato soup is sure to become a family favourite.

SERVES 4 ❄

Syns per serving
Original: 7
Green: Free

Preparation time 5 minutes
Cooking time 15 minutes

Fry Light

1 onion, peeled and finely chopped

2 sticks celery, trimmed and finely chopped

2 garlic cloves, peeled and finely chopped

1 litre/1¾ pints chicken stock made with Bovril (or vegetable stock made with Vecon)

4 ripe tomatoes, deseeded and finely chopped

200g/7oz cooked brown or white basmati rice

400g/14oz fresh or frozen peas

salt and freshly ground black pepper

To garnish
chopped herbs

1. Spray a saucepan with Fry Light and place over a medium heat. Add the onion, celery and garlic and stir-fry for 2–3 minutes. Add the stock and tomatoes and bring to the boil.

2. Reduce the heat to medium and cook for 5–6 minutes. Add the rice and peas and season well. Bring back to the boil and cook for 3–4 minutes, until the vegetables are cooked through. Remove from the heat and serve immediately, garnished with chopped fresh herbs of your choice.

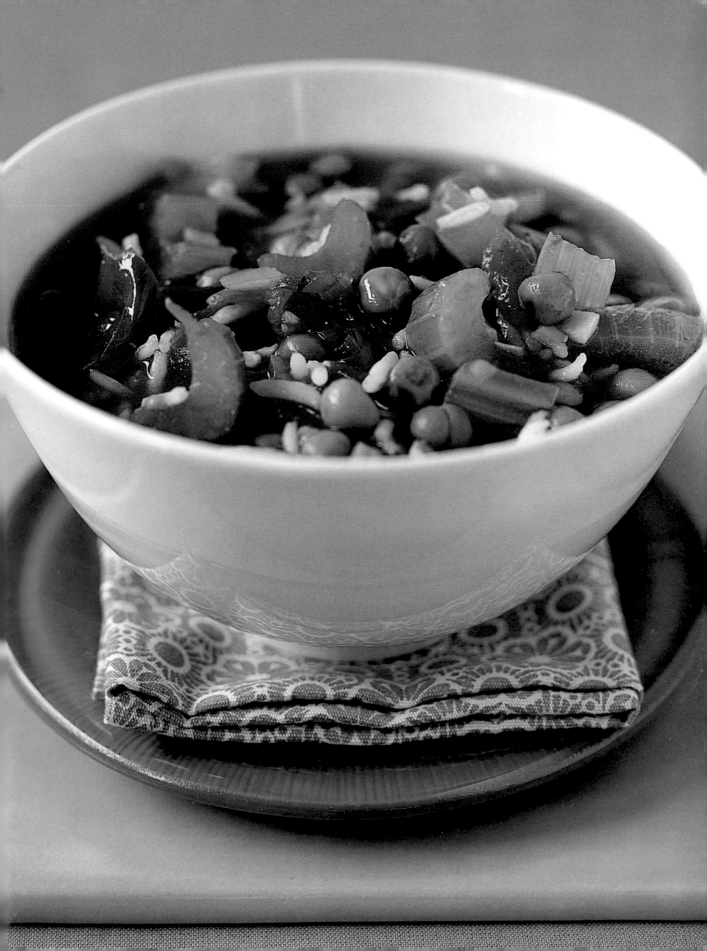

tomato, lentil and root vegetable soup

Garlic, ginger and curry powder add warmth to this colourful, satisfying soup. It would make a great supper on a winter's night.

SERVES 4 ⓥ ❋

Syns per serving
Original: 6
Green: Free

Preparation time 10 minutes
Cooking time about 20 minutes

Fry Light

1 onion, peeled and finely chopped

2 garlic cloves, peeled and crushed

1 tsp peeled and finely grated ginger

2 sticks celery, trimmed and finely chopped

1 large potato, peeled and cut into 1cm/½in dice

1 large carrot, peeled and cut into 1cm/½in dice

600ml/1 pint boiling water or vegetable stock made with Vecon

1 tbsp mild curry powder

125g/4½oz dried red lentils, rinsed and drained

600ml/1 pint passata

salt and freshly ground black pepper

1. Spray a large saucepan with Fry Light and place over a high heat. Add the onion, garlic, ginger, celery, potato and carrot and stir-fry for 1–2 minutes.

2. Add the remaining ingredients, except the seasoning, and bring to the boil. Cover and simmer gently for 15–20 minutes or until the lentils are cooked. Season well and serve immediately.

hot and sour seafood soup

Here's just the thing for a chilly evening – this light and flavoursome soup is fragrant, warm and comforting.

SERVES 4 ❋

Syns per serving
Original: Free
Green: 4

Preparation time 10 minutes
Cooking time about 10 minutes

1.2 litres/2 pints chicken stock made with Bovril

4 kaffir lime leaves

1 tsp peeled and finely grated ginger

1 red chilli, deseeded and finely sliced

1 tbsp finely chopped lemongrass

300g/11oz button mushrooms, halved

250g/9oz baby spinach leaves

300g/11oz cooked, peeled tiger prawns

juice of 1 lemon

salt and freshly ground black pepper

1. Place the stock, lime leaves, ginger, chilli and lemongrass into a saucepan and bring to the boil. Add the mushrooms, reduce the heat to a gentle simmer and cook for 2–3 minutes.

2. Add the spinach and prawns and simmer for a further 2–3 minutes until heated through.

3. Remove from the heat, add the lemon juice, season to taste and serve immediately, ladled into warmed bowls.

chilled yogurt and cucumber soup

This light and refreshing soup is the perfect food for a hot summer's day lunch. What's more, it's prepared in minutes and requires no cooking!

SERVES 4 Ⓥ

Syns per serving
Original: Free
Green: Free

Preparation time 5 minutes

2 large cucumbers

4 spring onions, trimmed and finely chopped

6 tbsp chopped mint leaves

500ml/18fl oz iced water

400g/14oz very low fat natural yogurt

2 tbsp raspberry vinegar

1 tsp sweet paprika or cayenne pepper

a pinch of ground cumin

salt and freshly ground black pepper

To garnish
very finely chopped mint leaves

1. Peel and halve the cucumbers lengthways. Using a small spoon, remove the seeds and discard. Chop the cucumber roughly and place in a food processor with the spring onions, mint and iced water. Blend until smooth.

2. Add the yogurt, vinegar, paprika (or cayenne pepper) and cumin, season well and blend again until smooth. Transfer to a bowl, cover and chill until required. Serve garnished with the chopped mint.

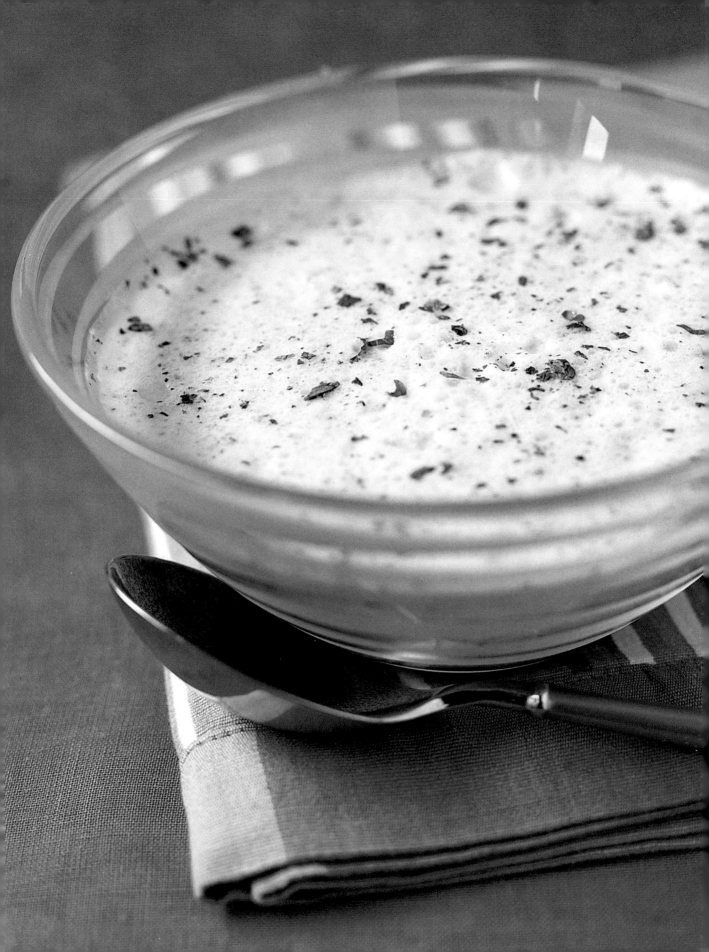

quick chicken noodle soup

This soup is an excellent choice as a starter for a heavier meal. It's also a good way of using up any leftover cooked chicken you may have.

SERVES 4 ✱

Syns per serving
Original: 2½
Green: 4½

Preparation time 5 minutes
Cooking time about 12 minutes

Fry Light

½ small onion, peeled and finely diced

1 garlic clove, peeled and finely diced

750ml/1¼ pints chicken stock made with Bovril

50g/2oz dried vermicelli or thin noodles

200g/7oz cooked chicken breasts, skinless and boneless

4 tbsp finely chopped flat-leaf parsley

salt and freshly ground black pepper

1. Spray a large, non-stick frying pan with Fry Light and place over a medium heat. Add the diced onion and garlic and gently stir-fry for 1–2 minutes.

2. Add the chicken stock and vermicelli or noodles and bring to the boil. Cover, reduce the heat to low and cook gently for 6–8 minutes until the vermicelli or noodles are cooked through.

3. Meanwhile, shred the chicken and add to the soup with the parsley and cook for 2–3 minutes or until piping hot. Season to taste and ladle into warmed bowls to serve.

watercress and leek soup

A perfect choice for those with milder tastes, this light soup allows the subtle flavours to come through.

SERVES 4 ❋

Syns per serving
Original: 1½
Green: Free

Preparation time 6–8 minutes
Cooking time about 15 minutes

Fry Light

4 leeks, white parts only, very thinly sliced

2 garlic cloves, peeled and finely chopped

1 large potato, peeled and cut into 1cm/½in dice

110g/4oz watercress, finely chopped

1 litre/1¾ pints chicken stock made with Bovril (or vegetable stock made with Vecon)

salt and freshly ground black pepper

To serve

very low fat natural fromage frais

1. Spray a non-stick saucepan with Fry Light and place over a medium heat. Add the leeks, garlic and potato and stir-fry for 2–3 minutes.

2. Add the watercress and stock and bring to the boil. Cover and cook gently for 10–12 minutes or until the potatoes are tender. Season well.

3. Using a blender or an electric hand-held processor, blend the soup until smooth. Ladle the soup into warmed bowls and serve with a dollop of fromage frais in the centre of each.

cabbage, carrot
and potato fritters

These versatile vegetable fritters make a great snack on their own, but would be equally good served as a main course accompaniment.

SERVES 4 ⓥ ❋

Syns per serving
Original: 2
Green: Free

Preparation time 6–8 minutes
Cooking time 25 minutes

For the tomato sauce

2 garlic cloves, peeled and chopped

200g can chopped tomatoes

1 tsp artificial sweetener

4 tbsp finely chopped basil leaves

salt and freshly ground black pepper

For the fritters

200g/7oz roughly grated potatoes

200g/7oz roughly grated carrots

200g/7oz finely shredded cabbage

1 spring onion, trimmed and finely sliced

1 tsp ground cumin

1 tsp ground coriander

1 tsp chilli powder

2 eggs, lightly beaten

Fry Light

To serve

very low fat natural yogurt

1. To make the tomato sauce, place the garlic, chopped tomatoes, sweetener and basil leaves in a small saucepan. Bring to the boil, then reduce the heat to low, cover and simmer gently for 15–20 minutes. Season well and remove from the heat. Leave to cool.

2. Meanwhile, make the fritters by mixing together all the ingredients, except the Fry Light, until thoroughly combined. Lightly spray a large, non-stick frying pan with Fry Light and place over a medium to high heat.

3. Working in batches, drop tablespoonfuls of the mixture onto the hot pan and flatten slightly with the back of a spoon. Cook for 3–4 minutes on each side, until golden. Remove with a slotted spoon and transfer to individual plates and serve with the tomato sauce and yogurt on the side.

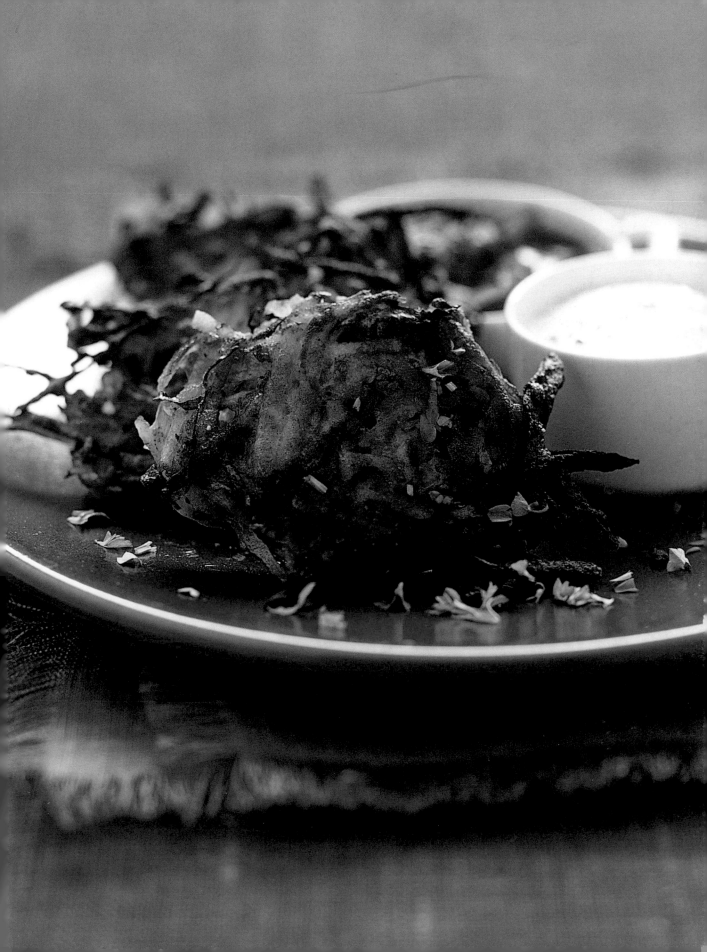

individual chive and mushroom quiches

These quiches have a delicious filling topped with a cheesy layer that sets when baked; they're low in Syns too! Enjoy them served straight from the oven.

MAKES 4 Ⓥ ❄

Syns per serving
Original: 3
Green: 3

Preparation time 10 minutes
Cooking time 15–20 minutes

Fry Light

4 spring onions, trimmed and finely sliced

2 garlic cloves, peeled and finely chopped

110g/4oz mushrooms, roughly chopped

freshly ground black pepper

2 x 25g/1oz sheets of filo pastry (thawed if frozen)

1 egg, beaten

2 tbsp Quark soft cheese

2 tbsp very low fat natural fromage frais

4 tbsp finely chopped chives

2 tbsp finely grated Parmesan cheese

2 cherry tomatoes, halved

To serve
tomato and mixed leaf salad

1. Preheat the oven to 200°C/Gas 6. Heat a large, non-stick frying pan over a high heat and spray with Fry Light. Add the spring onion and garlic and stir-fry for 3–4 minutes until lightly browned. Add the mushrooms and continue to cook over a high heat for 4–5 minutes until all the liquid has been absorbed. Season well with pepper and set aside.

2. Place the filo sheets next to each other on a clean work surface and cut each into six equal-sized pieces (giving you 12 pieces of filo pastry in all).

3. Lay one piece of pastry in the base of each of four 10cm/4in non-stick Yorkshire pudding tins. Brush with a little bit of the egg and lay another piece on top of it at a slightly different angle. Brush again with the egg and top with the remaining pastry to form a pastry 'shell'. Spoon the mushroom mixture into the pastry shells.

4. Mix together the remaining egg with the Quark, fromage frais, chives and Parmesan. Season with pepper and spoon this mixture over the mushroom mixture. Top each quiche with a halved cherry tomato and bake in the oven for 15–20 minutes until lightly browned and just set. Serve warm with a tomato and mixed leaf salad.

potato and red pepper squares

These 'frittata' squares make a great Green day snack or lunchbox filler. Enjoy them any time, anywhere!

SERVES 4 Ⓥ ❄

Syns per serving
Original: 3½
Green: Free

Preparation time 5 minutes
Cooking time 20–25 minutes

Fry Light
400g/14oz peeled and boiled potatoes
6 spring onions, trimmed and finely sliced
200g/7oz roasted red peppers, cut into small pieces
4 tbsp finely chopped parsley
salt and freshly ground black pepper
4 eggs, lightly beaten

1. Preheat the oven to 220°C/Gas 7. Lightly spray a 20cm/8in square non-stick baking tin with Fry Light. Cut the potatoes into small dice.

2. Mix together the potatoes, spring onions, peppers and parsley. Season well and spread over the prepared baking tin. Pour over the eggs and place in the oven and bake for 20–25 minutes or until set and golden. Remove from the oven and allow to cool before cutting into squares. Serve at room temperature.

stuffed garlic mushrooms
with spinach

Here is a simple-yet-tasty starter that makes the most of the meaty texture of mushrooms. It's great served hot with couscous, rice or a salad.

SERVES 4 Ⓥ

Syns per serving
Original: 3
Green: 3

Preparation time 5 minutes
Cooking time about 25 minutes

8 large flat field mushrooms, cleaned and stalks removed

Fry Light

salt and freshly ground black pepper

2 garlic cloves, peeled and crushed

300g/11oz baby spinach leaves

a pinch of grated nutmeg

50g/2oz Parmesan cheese, grated

1. Preheat the grill to medium. Spray the mushrooms all over with Fry Light and place on a grill rack, cap-side up, and grill gently for 5–6 minutes, then turn them over, season well and grill for another 5 minutes or until they start weeping black juice. Remove from the grill. Turn up the grill to high.

2. Spray a large, non-stick frying pan with Fry Light and place over a high heat. Add the garlic and spinach and stir-fry for 4–5 minutes or until the spinach has just wilted. Add the nutmeg, season well and divide this mixture into eight and top the mushrooms with it.

3. Sprinkle over the cheese and place under the hot grill for 2–3 minutes or until melted and bubbling. Serve immediately with couscous, rice or a salad.

pink peppercorn and smoked salmon pâté

This easy-to-prepare smoked salmon pâté makes a great starter or healthy snack on an Original day. Just dip in and enjoy!

SERVES 4 ❄

Syns per serving
Original: Free
Green: 9

Preparation time 5 minutes
Cooking time 2–3 minutes

Fry Light
6 spring onions, trimmed and finely sliced
500g/1lb 2oz smoked salmon
250g/9oz Quark soft cheese
2 tbsp dried pink peppercorns
2 tsp finely grated lemon zest
4 tbsp finely chopped dill

To serve
assortment of vegetable crudités, e.g. carrot sticks, celery sticks, sliced peppers, radishes

1. Spray a large, non-stick frying pan with Fry Light and sauté the spring onions for 2–3 minutes until softened.

2. Transfer the spring onions to a food processor and add the remaining ingredients. Blend until smooth. Transfer to a serving dish and chill the pâté until ready to serve with a variety of vegetable crudités to dip into it.

smoked salmon
and cucumber rolls

This simple-yet-elegant dinner party starter will wow your guests yet only you need ever know just how quick they are to prepare.

SERVES 4

Syns per serving
Original: Free
Green: 6

Preparation time 10 minutes

12 x 25g/1oz slices of smoked salmon

1 cucumber, peeled, deseeded and cut into thin matchsticks

½ small red pepper, deseeded and cut into thin slivers

a small handful of mint leaves, chopped

1 tsp finely grated lemon zest

freshly ground black pepper

To garnish
finely sliced lemon peel

1. Separate the smoked salmon slices and lay them out on a clean, flat work surface.

2. In a bowl, mix together the cucumber, red pepper, mint and lemon zest. Season with the black pepper.

3. Divide this mixture onto the salmon slices in small mounds and then roll up the slices to enclose the filling. Serve immediately, garnished with the lemon peel.

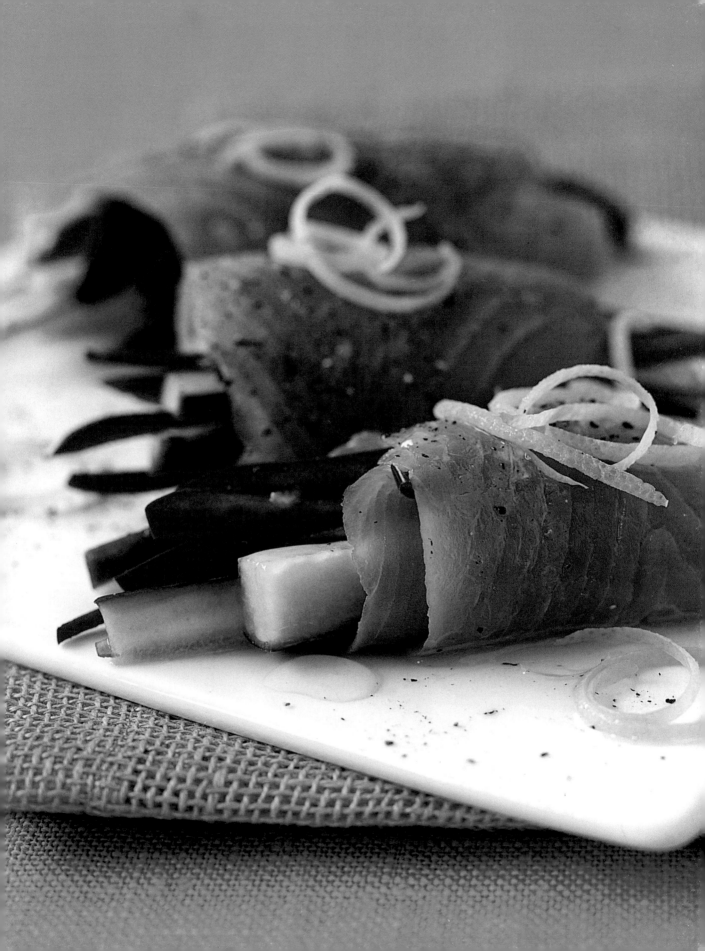

ginger
prawn cakes

Prepared in just minutes, these succulent, spicy fish cakes are a wonderful way to start any meal.

SERVES 4 ✻

Syns per serving
Original: Free
Green: 6

Preparation time 10 minutes
plus chilling

Cooking time 5–6 minutes

For the cakes

400g/14oz peeled raw tiger prawns

200g/7oz extra-lean pork mince

1 red chilli, deseeded and finely chopped

2 spring onions, trimmed and finely sliced

1 tsp peeled and finely grated ginger

3 tbsp chopped coriander leaves

1 tbsp finely chopped mint leaves

1 tsp finely grated lime zest

salt and freshly ground black pepper

Fry Light

To serve

mixed salad leaves

1. To make the cakes, place all the ingredients, except the seasoning and Fry Light, in a food processor and process until well blended. Season well and transfer to a bowl. Cover and chill for 1–2 hours or overnight if time permits.

2. When ready to cook, divide the mixture into 12 portions and form each one into a cake. Lightly spray some Fry Light into a shallow, non-stick frying pan and place over a medium heat. Add the cakes into the pan and fry for 2–3 minutes on each side until lightly browned.

3. To serve, line four plates with mixed salad leaves and divide the cakes between them. Serve immediately.

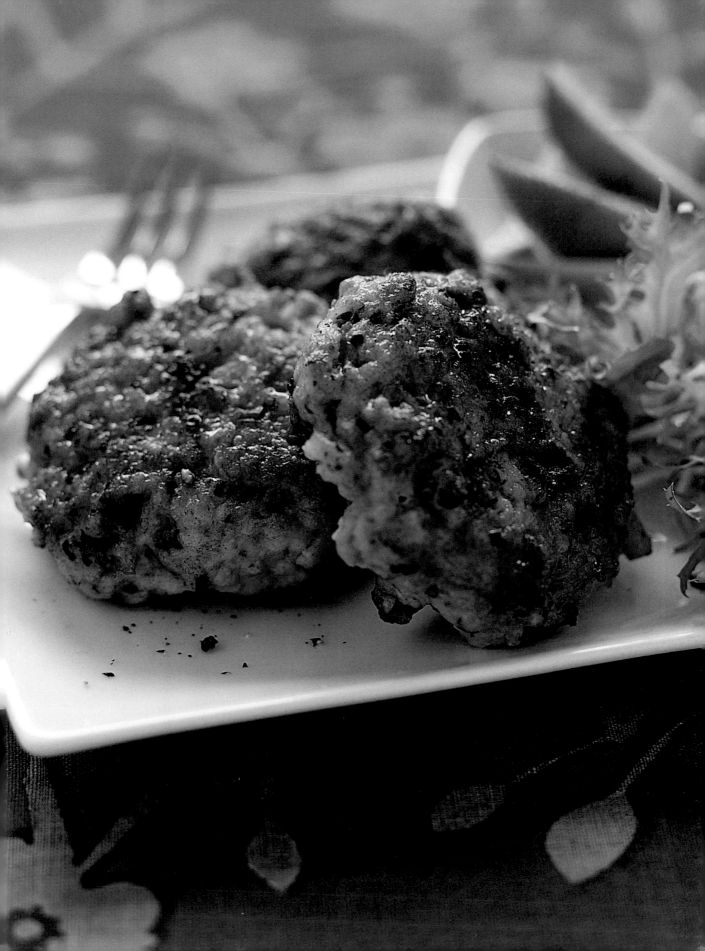

smoked trout florentine
with dill hollandaise sauce

A simple dish of trout fillets served on a bed of creamy spinach and drizzled with hollandaise sauce. Salmon or mackerel would make good alternatives to the trout.

SERVES 4

Syns per serving
Original: Free
Green: 8

Preparation time 10 minutes
Cooking time 3–4 minutes

For the sauce

4 tbsp Quark soft cheese

8 tbsp very low fat natural fromage frais

60ml/2fl oz hot chicken stock made with Bovril

6 tbsp finely chopped dill

2 tbsp finely chopped chives

1 tsp English mustard powder

salt and freshly ground black pepper

For the trout

Fry Light

2 garlic cloves, peeled and finely chopped

400g/14oz baby spinach leaves

4 x 110g/4oz hot-smoked trout fillets

1. Make the hollandaise sauce by placing all the ingredients, except the seasoning, into a blender and process until smooth. Season to taste, transfer to a bowl and set aside.

2. Spray a large, non-stick frying pan with Fry Light. Place over a medium heat and add the garlic and spinach. Stir and cook for 3–4 minutes or until the spinach has just wilted. Season well and remove from the heat.

3. To serve, divide the spinach mixture between four warmed plates in neat mounds and top with the trout fillets. Spoon over the sauce and serve immediately.

devilled chicken wings

Finger-lickin' good, these devilled chicken wings will have you coming back for more. They are great for cooking on the 'barbie'.

SERVES 4 ✳

Syns per serving
Original: 1
Green: 5

Preparation time 5 minutes plus marinating
Cooking time 15–20 minutes

600g/1lb 6oz large chicken wings, skinned

For the marinade
1 small onion, peeled and finely diced
1 tbsp clear honey
2 tbsp Worcestershire sauce
1 tbsp paprika
2 tbsp passata
1 tsp cayenne pepper
1 tsp ground cumin
salt and freshly ground black pepper

To serve
lemon wedges

1. Place the chicken wings in a large shallow bowl in a single layer.

2. Mix together all the marinade ingredients, except the seasoning, and pour over the chicken. Season and mix well to coat the chicken evenly. Cover and leave to marinate for 1–2 hours or overnight if time permits.

3. Preheat the grill to medium-hot. Place the chicken wings in a single layer on a grill pan and grill for 15–20 minutes, turning once, or until the chicken is cooked through. Remove from the grill and serve the chicken either warm or at room temperature with lemon wedges.

chicken
and bacon brochettes

Succulent chicken breast pieces, flavoured with lemon and rosemary, wrapped in bacon and then grilled to perfection. Simple!

SERVES 4 ❅

Syns per serving
Original: Free
Green: 15½

Preparation time 10 minutes
Cooking time about 10 minutes

4 large skinless chicken breasts, each cut into 8 bite-sized chunks

finely grated zest and juice of 1 lemon

1 tsp finely chopped rosemary leaves

salt and freshly ground black pepper

16 rashers of lean bacon, each cut into 2 pieces

16 cherry tomatoes

Fry Light

To serve
chopped parsley
mixed green salad

1. Place the chicken in a bowl and toss with the lemon zest, juice and rosemary. Season well.

2. To assemble the skewers, wrap each piece of chicken with a piece of bacon – you will end up with 32 wrapped chicken pieces. Onto each of eight metal skewers, thread a cherry tomato, then four chicken pieces and then another cherry tomato.

3. Preheat the grill to medium-hot. Lightly spray the skewers with Fry Light and grill for 8–10 minutes, turning once, or until the chicken is cooked through and the bacon is lightly browned. Garnish with chopped parsley and serve immediately with a mixed green salad.

ham
and egg 'soufflés'

A step up from a ham omelette, these individual soufflés would also make a lovely light lunch, served with a fresh crisp salad.

SERVES 4
Syns per serving
With Parmesan
Original: 1
Green: 3
Without Parmesan
Original: Free
Green: 2

Preparation time 10 minutes
Cooking time 12–15 minutes

Fry Light
2 eggs, separated
110g/4oz lean ham, finely chopped
1 tbsp finely chopped tarragon
4 tbsp finely chopped flat-leaf parsley
1 tbsp finely chopped chives
salt and freshly ground black pepper
2 tbsp finely grated Parmesan cheese (optional)

1. Preheat the oven to 200°C/Gas 6. Lightly spray four individual ovenproof soufflé dishes with Fry Light and place them on a baking sheet.

2. In a bowl, beat the egg yolks until pale and fluffy. Stir in the chopped ham and herbs. Season well.

3. In a separate bowl, whisk the egg whites until softly peaked and, using a metal spoon, fold into the ham mixture. Spoon this mixture into the prepared dishes. Sprinkle over the Parmesan cheese, if using, and place in the oven and bake for 12–15 minutes until risen and golden. Remove from the oven and serve immediately.

no more yo-yo dieting for Sarah

Sarah Bennett lives in Goudhurst, Kent, with her husband Tim, their son Sam and Sarah's daughter Emma. She ended a 14-year struggle with her weight after it reached 13st 3lb, by losing 3st 10lb with Slimming World.

Sarah Bennett found a healthy way to slim and stay trim after 14 years of yo-yo diets and ill health. And she feels so passionate about how much it has helped her that she decided to help others as well – by becoming a Slimming World Consultant.

Her weight began to climb with her first pregnancy and continued to worsen through a series of family tragedies, including the deaths of her son, father and brother, the break-up of her first marriage and debilitating bouts of irritable bowel syndrome (IBS).

Even new happiness failed to halt her rising weight and, after she met and married sales manager Tim and gave birth to Sam, the family enjoyed cosy home-cooked meals and lots of chocolate.

'I put on weight from comfort eating because of my circumstances but once it becomes a habit, it's so hard to break,' says Sarah. 'If it hadn't been for our Christmas photographs in 2003 I might have stayed big forever. I couldn't believe the woman with the big puffy face was really me. Shortly afterwards I found myself in the changing room of a plus-sized shop, fitting into a size 20. I was horrified and resolved there and then to do whatever it took to get back to a healthy weight.'

A friend guided Sarah towards a local Slimming World group and she knew straight away she would keep her resolution. Less than a year later, Sarah had swapped her size 20 clothes for a wardrobe of size 10 outfits and vowed never to return to yo-yo dieting. She said: 'As soon as I looked at the Food Optimising books I was confident it would work perfectly, despite my restricted diet. Rice milk, which I put on cereal, and soya milk, which I use for everything from coffee to omelettes, are both Healthy Extra choices on both Green and Original days, and gluten-free rice and corn pastas are Free on Green days.

'My husband loves to Food Optimise, too, and loves vegetarian options such as ratatouille. Basic dishes can be adapted in so many ways. A tin of tomatoes, garlic and onion cooked in a little olive oil is wonderful with pasta. You can add all sorts of things such as mushrooms, courgettes and aubergines. People don't even notice there is no meat on the plate!

'And we always enjoy the most delicious soups on a Monday. We enjoy six or seven vegetables with our Sunday roast because we all love them so much and anything left over goes into a soup on Monday because it's incredibly good and very easy!'

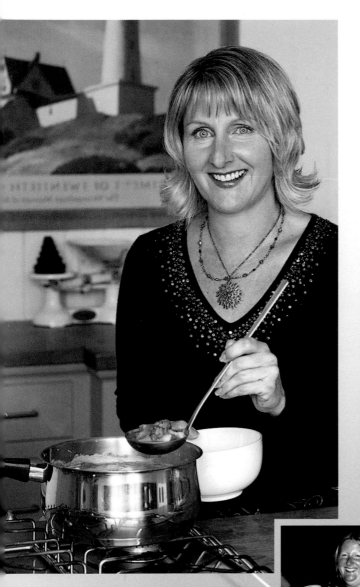

make the past work
for you,
not against you

If you've ever tried to lose weight before, and failed – or lost and then regained weight – how do you view that time? As a failure? A sign that you are weak or that you have some unseen, fatal flaw? There can be little surprise, then, when all your good intentions seem to crumble before you've had the chance to make a change. Yesterday, last week, last year . . . none of these things are important. Decide today that the past can highlight potential pitfalls. Learn from them. Then look to the future and focus on tomorrow's you.

"I'm a veteran of several slimming clubs and this was the first time I'd ever been encouraged to get to know my fellow slimmers. I think Slimming World was designed with me in mind – and I love the way Free Food works because it means you never run out of meal options."

snacks and salads

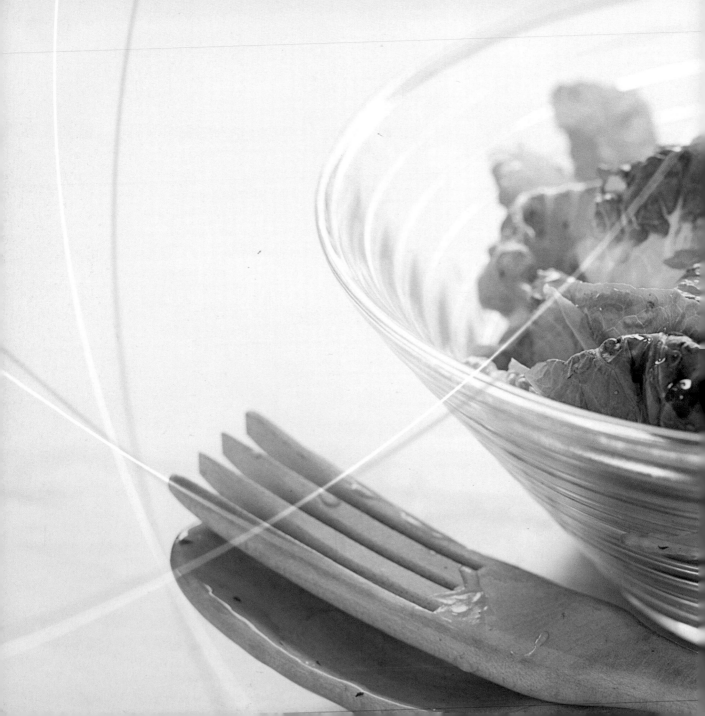

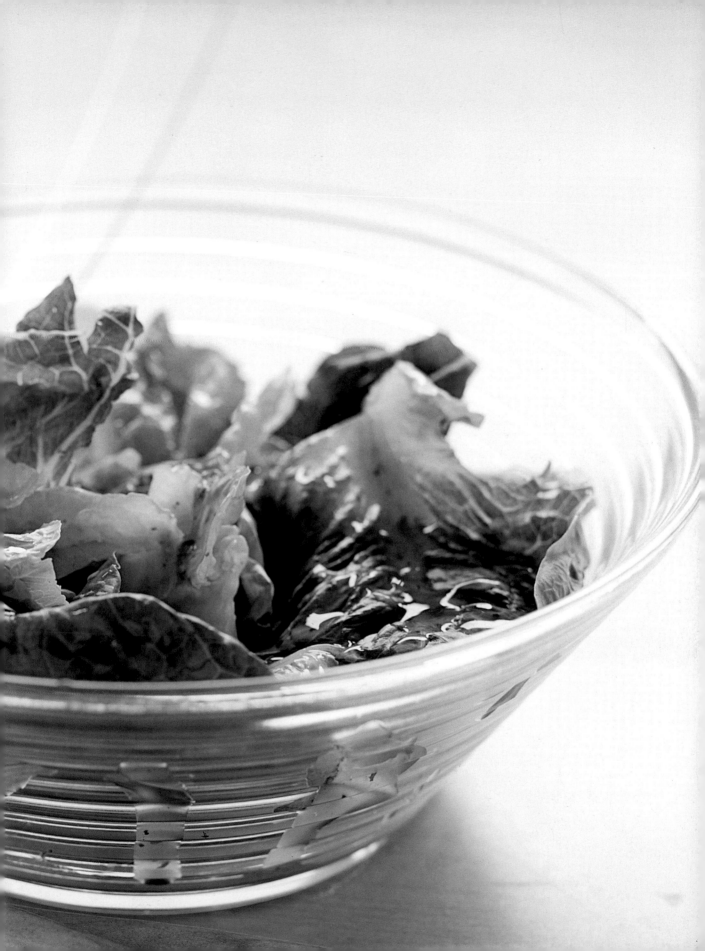

pimenton potato wedges
with coriander and tomato dip

Potatoes are a real comfort food and this recipe is no exception. It makes a fabulous snack any time.

SERVES 4 Ⓥ

Syns per serving
Original: 8½
Green: 2½

Preparation time 10 minutes
Cooking time 15–20 minutes

For the dip

400g/14oz very low fat natural fromage frais

1 garlic clove, peeled and finely grated

finely grated zest of 1 lemon

6 tbsp finely chopped coriander leaves

2 ripe tomatoes, deseeded and finely chopped

salt and freshly ground black pepper

For the wedges

4 large potatoes, unpeeled and cut into quarters

4 spring onions, trimmed and finely chopped

3 ripe plum tomatoes, finely chopped

2 red peppers, deseeded and very finely chopped

1 tbsp pimenton or mild paprika

1 tsp dried mixed herbs

salt and freshly ground black pepper

Fry Light

110g/4oz reduced fat mozzarella cheese

1. To make the dip, mix together the fromage frais, garlic, lemon zest, coriander and tomatoes. Season well and chill until ready to serve.

2. Preheat the oven to 220°C/Gas 7. Place the potatoes in a large saucepan of lightly salted boiling water, reduce the heat and simmer for 4–5 minutes. Drain thoroughly and when cool, scoop out the flesh from each quarter, leaving a 1cm/½in-thick layer. Discard the scooped-out potato (you can save it for another use, such as in a soup or as mash) and place the potato wedges, scooped side up, on a non-stick parchment-lined baking sheet.

3. In a bowl, mix together the spring onions, tomatoes, peppers, pimenton and dried mixed herbs. Season well and then spoon this mixture into the potato quarters and lightly spray with Fry Light. Top with the cheese and bake for 15–20 minutes or until crisp and golden. Serve immediately with the dip.

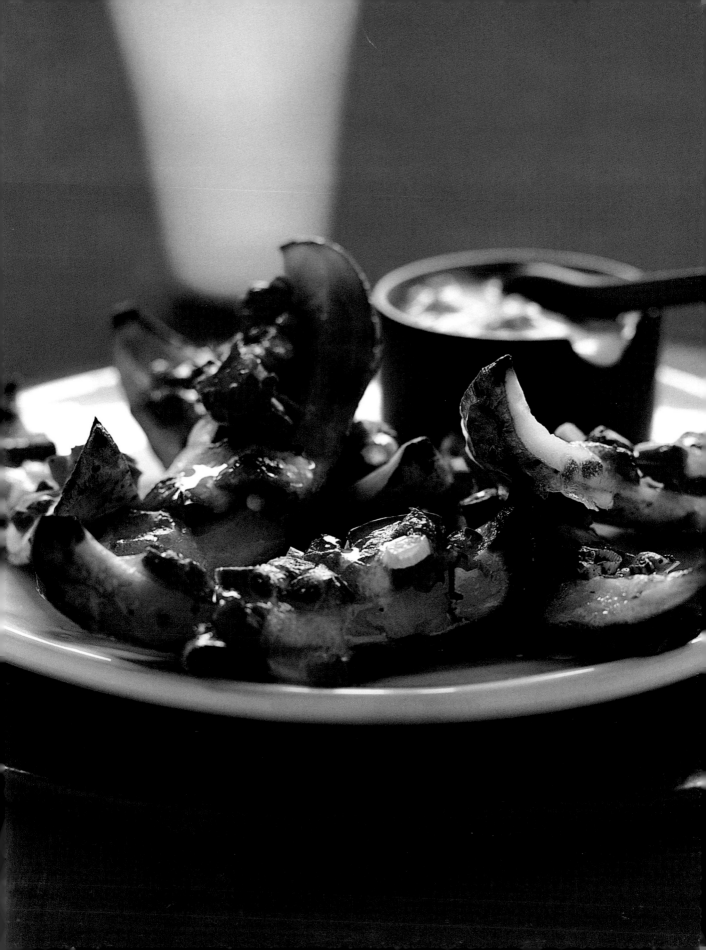

fresh herbed
omelette

Turn a humble omelette into a delicious simple snack in a matter of minutes by adding lots of fresh herbs.

MAKES 1 Ⓥ

Syns per serving
Original: 2
Green: Free

Preparation time 10 minutes
Cooking time 6–8 minutes

50g/2oz peeled and cooked potatoes, roughly diced

4 tbsp finely chopped chives

4 tbsp finely chopped dill

4 tbsp finely chopped flat-leaf parsley

2 tbsp very low fat natural fromage frais

2 eggs

salt and freshly ground black pepper

Fry Light

To serve
crisp green salad
chopped chives (optional)

1. Place the cooked potatoes and chives, dill and flat-leaf parsley in a bowl and stir in the fromage frais. Set aside.

2. Crack the eggs into a mixing bowl, add seasoning and 2 teaspoons of water. Beat lightly.

3. Spray a non-stick frying pan with Fry Light and place over a medium heat. When hot, pour in the egg mixture, tilting and rotating the pan to cover the base evenly. Quickly stir the eggs with a fork as they start to set and gently lift the edges so that any liquid egg can flow underneath.

4. When the underside of the omelette has started to set, spoon over the potato mixture evenly and then, using a spatula, carefully fold the omelette over. Cook for 1–2 minutes or until cooked to your liking and then carefully slide out onto a warmed plate. Serve immediately with a crisp, green salad. Garnish with chopped chives if desired.

spiced egg
toasts

This is scrambled eggs on toast – but not as you currently know it!

SERVES 4 Ⓥ
Syns per serving
Original: 3
Green: 3

Preparation time 5–6 minutes
Cooking time 6–8 minutes

6 eggs

1 onion, peeled and very finely chopped

1 red chilli, deseeded and finely sliced (optional)

4 tbsp very finely chopped flat-leaf parsley

1 plum tomato, deseeded and finely diced

¼ tsp ground cumin

¼ tsp ground coriander

salt and freshly ground black pepper

Fry Light

To serve
4 slices wholemeal toast from a small 400g loaf

1. In a large mixing bowl, beat the eggs lightly. Stir in the onion, chilli, flat-leaf parsley, tomato, cumin and coriander. Season well and mix to combine.

2. Spray a non-stick frying pan with Fry Light and place over a medium heat. Add the egg mixture, stir and reduce the heat. Let the mixture cook undisturbed for 2–3 minutes and then, using a wooden spoon, stir and cook gently for 3–4 minutes until the eggs start to scramble and set or until cooked to your liking. Remove from the heat.

3. Divide the egg mixture between the four slices of wholemeal toast and serve immediately.

ratatouille jackets

Enliven a jacket spud with a generous topping of tasty home-made ratatouille and enjoy it either as a snack or as a light lunch served with salad.

SERVES 4 Ⓥ

Syns per serving
Original: 6
Green: Free

Preparation time 10 minutes
Cooking time about 10 minutes

4 large baking potatoes
Fry Light
Sea salt

For the ratatouille
1 garlic clove, peeled and chopped
4 spring onions, trimmed and chopped
1 red pepper, deseeded and cut into 1cm/½in dice
½ courgette, cut into 1cm/½in dice
¼ aubergine, cut into 1cm/½in dice
4 tbsp canned, chopped tomatoes
a large handful of flat-leaf parsley, roughly chopped
salt and freshly ground black pepper

1. Prick the baking potatoes all over with a skewer, spray with Fry Light and sprinkle with sea salt. Place in a microwave at the highest power and cook for 10–12 minutes or until tender.

2. Meanwhile, make the pan-fried ratatouille. Heat a large, non-stick frying pan, spray with Fry Light and add the garlic, spring onions, red pepper, courgette and aubergine. Cook over a high heat for 4–5 minutes, stirring often, until the vegetables start to brown at the edges. Stir in the tomatoes and continue to cook for 2–3 minutes. Stir in the flat-leaf parsley, remove from the heat and season well. (This can be made the night before and reheated quickly on the day in a frying pan.)

3. Serve the jacket potatoes, split in halves or quarters, with the ratatouille spooned over them.

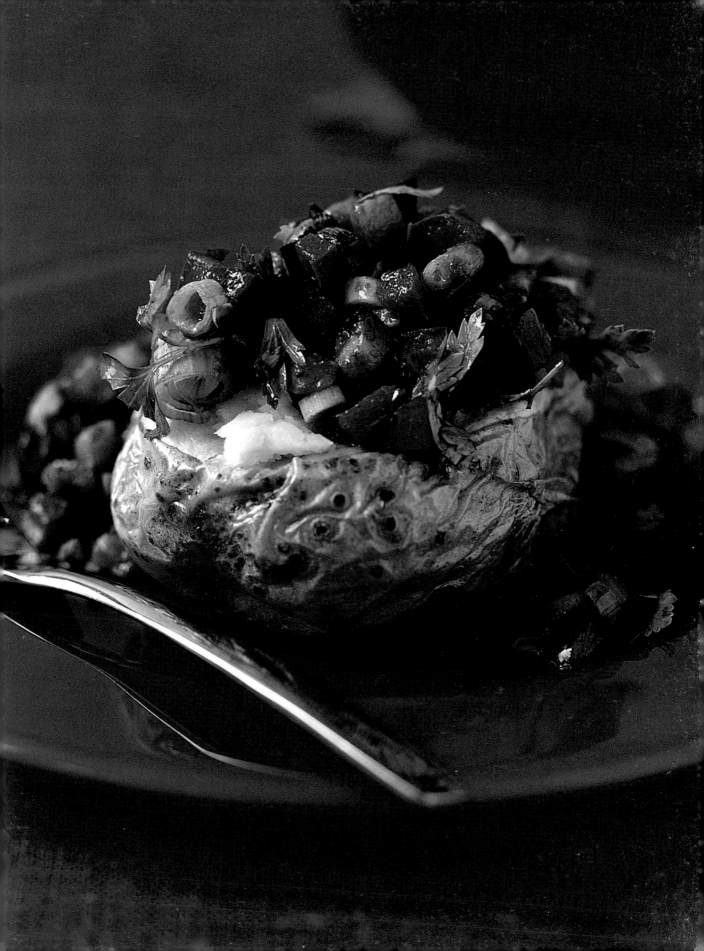

chicken
and egg wraps

Quick, tasty and Free on Slimming World's Original plan, these chicken and egg wraps will soon become a family favourite!

SERVES 4

Syns per serving
Original: Free
Green: 9½

Preparation time 10 minutes
Cooking time about 20 minutes

For the filling
Fry Light

4 spring onions, peeled and chopped

2 garlic cloves, peeled and chopped

1 small carrot, peeled and diced

1 stick celery, trimmed and diced

3 cooked chicken breasts, thinly shredded

4 plum tomatoes, chopped

2 tbsp passata

1 tbsp finely chopped basil

salt and freshly ground black pepper

For the wraps
8 eggs, lightly beaten

4 tbsp chopped mixed herbs

To serve
green salad

1. To make the filling, spray a large saucepan with Fry Light. Place over a high heat and add the spring onions, garlic, carrot, celery and chicken. Stir-fry for 3–4 minutes until the vegetables have softened and then add the tomatoes, passata and basil. Season and cook gently for 10 minutes or until the mixture is heated through.

2. Meanwhile, make the wraps. In a bowl, mix together the eggs and herbs. Season well and heat a non-stick frying pan over a medium heat. Spray with Fry Light and pour a quarter of the egg mixture into the pan. Swirl to cover the base and cook for 1–2 minutes on each side. Remove and set aside while you use up the rest of the egg mixture in the same way so that you end up with four egg 'wraps'.

3. To serve, divide the filling into four portions and spoon into the centre of each wrap. Roll up to enclose the filling and serve immediately with a crisp green salad.

quick
tex-mex tacos

A quick and healthy version of a much-loved snack. To make it Syn-free on the Original plan, replace the taco shells with large iceberg lettuce leaves, spoon the chicken mixture into the leaves, wrap and eat.

SERVES 4 ❀ (filling only)

Syns per serving
Original: 2½
Green: 12

Preparation time 6–8 minutes
Cooking time 6–8 minutes

Fry Light

2 garlic cloves, peeled and finely chopped

1 red onion, peeled, halved and thinly sliced

½ red pepper, deseeded and thinly sliced

1 tsp ground cumin

1 tsp mild paprika

4 tbsp canned, chopped tomatoes

3 cooked chicken breasts, skinned and thinly sliced

salt and freshly ground black pepper

4 taco shells

a handful of shredded iceberg lettuce leaves

1. Heat a large, non-stick frying pan sprayed with Fry Light. When hot add the garlic, red onion, red pepper, cumin, paprika, tomatoes and chicken, season well and stir-fry for 5–6 minutes, stirring and shaking the pan constantly until the mixture is hot and the vegetables are just tender.

2. Place the taco shells on a serving tray and line with the shredded iceberg lettuce. Spoon over the chicken mixture and serve the tacos immediately.

skillet 'pizzas'

The potato and egg base makes this a really filling snack. We've topped it with cherry tomatoes, but you could use chopped mushrooms, peppers or onions – the choice is yours!

SERVES 4 Ⓥ

Syns per serving
Original: 7
Green: Free

Preparation time 10 minutes
Cooking time about 15 minutes

Fry Light

800g/1lb 12oz peeled, boiled (for 6–7 minutes) and grated potatoes

1 small egg, lightly beaten

salt and freshly ground black pepper

For the topping

200g/7oz cherry tomatoes, halved or quartered

3 garlic cloves, peeled and crushed

a small handful of rocket leaves, chopped

1. Spray a 22cm/8½in non-stick skillet or frying pan with Fry Light. In a bowl, mix together the grated potatoes and egg. Season and spoon this mixture into the prepared skillet or frying pan, pressing down with the back of a spoon to make a flat base.

2. Place the skillet or frying pan over a medium heat and cook the 'pizza' base for 8–10 minutes.

3. Meanwhile, preheat the grill to medium-hot. Mix together the cherry tomatoes and garlic in a bowl, crushing them lightly with a fork. Spoon onto the top of the potato mixture and place under the grill for 3–4 minutes or until the mixture is bubbling and hot. Remove from the grill, scatter over the rocket leaves and serve straight from the pan.

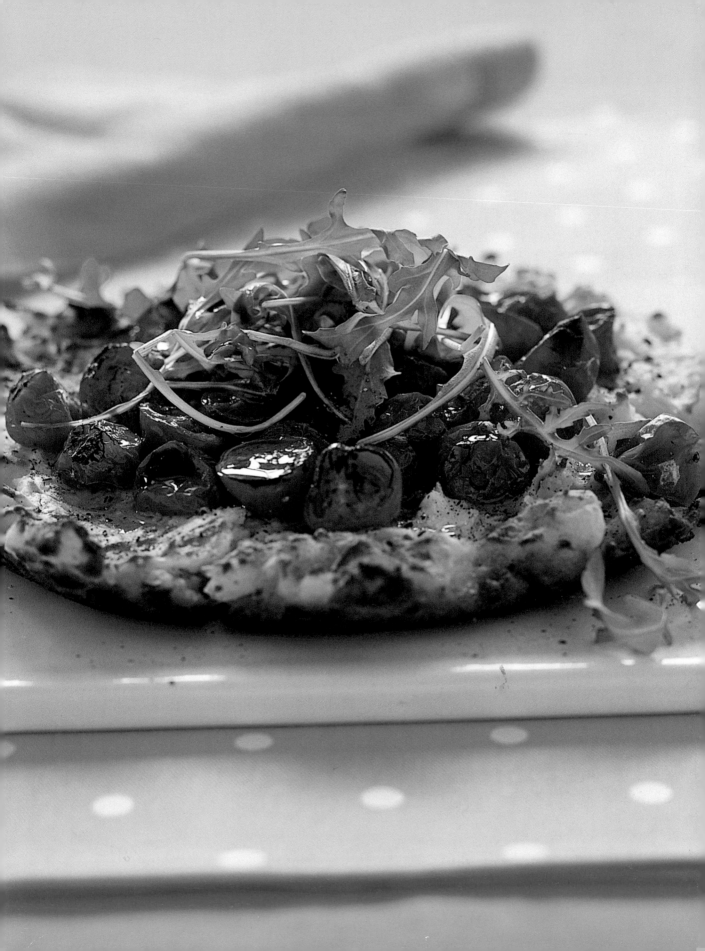

manhattan-style
burgers

Perfect summer barbecue fare, this quick and healthy burger will go down a storm with everyone.

SERVES 4 ❄ (burgers only)

Syns per serving
Original: Free
Green: 16

Preparation time 6–8 minutes
Cooking time about 10 minutes

500g/1lb 2oz extra-lean beef mince

500g/1lb 2oz extra-lean pork mince

2 garlic cloves, peeled and crushed

2 tbsp finely diced onion

1 tsp dried oregano

2 tbsp finely chopped parsley

salt and freshly ground black pepper

Fry Light

To serve

crisp green salad leaves, red onion rings, sliced tomatoes, gherkins

1. Place the mince in a bowl with the garlic, onion, dried oregano and parsley and season well. Using your fingers, combine the ingredients thoroughly and then divide the mixture into eight portions. Shape each portion into a thick 'burger' and spray them lightly with Fry Light.

2. Preheat the grill to medium-hot. Place the burgers on a grill rack and grill for 5 minutes on each side or until cooked to your liking. Remove from the grill and serve two burgers per portion together with crisp green salad leaves, red onion rings, sliced tomatoes and gherkins.

tomato, basil and mozzarella salad

This simple-yet-attractive salad combines juicy tomatoes with smooth mozzarella cheese. Add a few basil leaves and a drizzle of fat-free dressing and – Voila!

SERVES 4 Ⓥ

Syns per serving
Original: 2½
Green: 2½

Preparation time 5 minutes

6 plum tomatoes, cut into 1.5cm/¾in pieces
110g/4oz reduced fat mozzarella cheese, cut into 1cm/½in pieces
a large handful of basil leaves
6 tbsp fat-free salad dressing
salt and freshly ground black pepper

1. Place the tomatoes on a shallow serving platter or in a bowl. Scatter the mozzarella cheese over the tomatoes.

2. Roughly tear the basil leaves and scatter them over the tomato and mozzarella mixture.

3. Drizzle over the salad dressing, season well and toss thoroughly to mix. Serve immediately.

ten-minute beans and bangers

A warming, satisfying snack that's Free on the Green plan. Children will love it – if they get a look in, that is!

SERVES 4

Syns per serving
Original: 7½
Green: Free

Preparation time 2–3 minutes
Cooking time 7–8 minutes

Fry Light

8 Quorn sausages

400g can chopped tomatoes

a generous splash of Worcestershire sauce

a generous splash of dark soy sauce

1 tsp chopped fresh thyme

4 spring onions, trimmed and finely sliced

2 garlic cloves, peeled and crushed

1 tsp paprika

400g can cannellini beans, drained and rinsed

400g can butter beans, drained and rinsed

salt and freshly ground black pepper

1. Spray a large, non-stick frying pan with Fry Light and place over a medium heat. Cook the sausages for 2–3 minutes until they are lightly browned all over.

2. Add all the remaining ingredients and cook over a high heat for 4–5 minutes until bubbling. Season well, remove from the heat and serve immediately.

herbed chickpea and tabbouleh salad

A really quick salad to prepare, this one is packed full of colour and flavour. It's perfect for a lunchbox or picnic.

SERVES 4 Ⓥ

Syns per serving
Original: 9½
Green: ½

Preparation time 10 minutes

150g/5oz bulgur wheat

3 large oranges

1 red onion, peeled, roughly chopped or cut into rings

4 vine tomatoes, roughly chopped

1 cucumber, roughly chopped

200g can chickpeas, drained

a small bunch of coriander leaves, finely chopped

a small bunch of mint leaves, finely chopped

a small bunch of flat-leaf parsley, finely chopped

For the dressing
juice of 1 orange

juice of 1 lemon

1 tsp ground cumin

1 tsp ground ginger

1 tsp garlic granules or 1 garlic clove, peeled and crushed

salt and freshly ground black pepper

To serve
lettuce leaves

herbs to garnish (optional)

1. Prepare the bulgur wheat according to the packet instructions and set aside. When ready, place the wheat in a sieve, squeeze dry and transfer to a wide bowl.

2. Peel the oranges with a sharp knife and cut into segments, over a bowl, saving any juices.

3. Add the orange segments, red onion, tomatoes, cucumber, chickpeas and herbs to the bulgur wheat and toss to mix well.

4. To make the dressing, mix all the ingredients together with the saved orange juice, season and pour over the salad ingredients. Toss to mix well.

5. To serve, arrange the lettuce leaves across four serving plates and pile on the salad, garnishing with fresh herbs if desired.

red chicory, red onion and watercress salad

Here's a simple salad that's great either on its own or eaten as a main course accompaniment.

SERVES 4 ⓥ

Syns per serving
Original: Free
Green: Free

Preparation time 5 minutes

2 heads of red chicory

2 red onions, peeled, halved and thinly sliced

225g/8oz watercress

6 tbsp fat-free salad dressing

salt and freshly ground black pepper

1. Wash and separate the chicory leaves and place in a large salad bowl with the red onion and watercress.

2. Drizzle over the dressing and toss to mix well.

3. Season to taste and serve immediately.

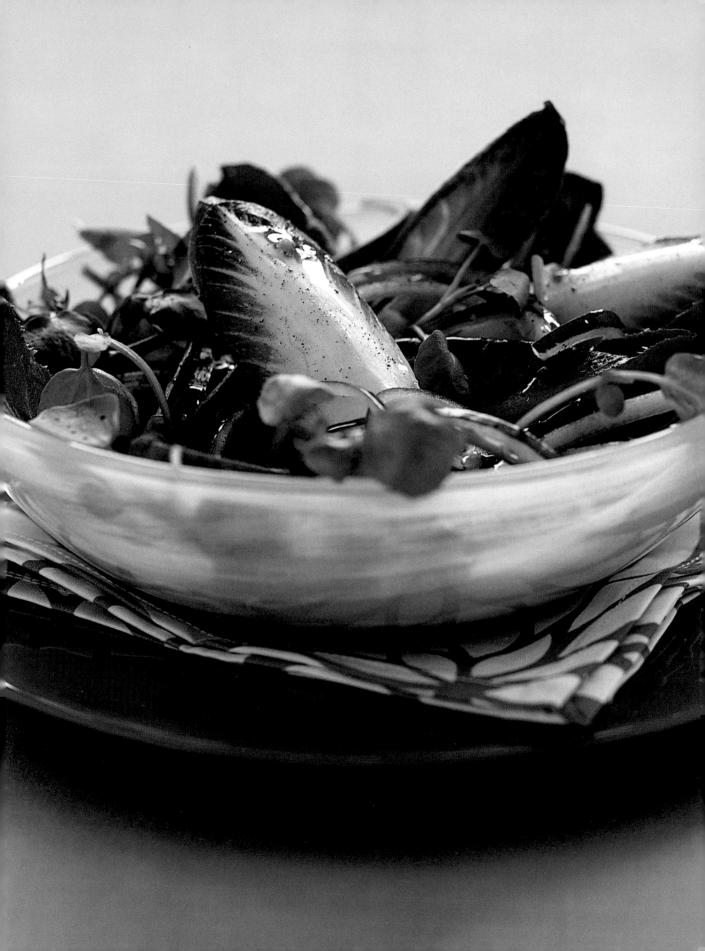

mixed bean
and pasta salad

Green beans, carrots and spring onions add crunch to this filling pasta salad, which is simply tossed in a sweet-and-sour dressing.

SERVES 4 Ⓥ

Syns per serving
Original: 5½
Green: Free

Preparation time 10 minutes
Cooking time 2–3 minutes

200g/7oz green beans, trimmed and halved widthways

2 carrots, peeled and cut into thin matchsticks

salt and freshly ground black pepper

400g can mixed beans, drained and rinsed

110g/4oz cherry tomatoes, halved

3 spring onions, trimmed and finely sliced

110g/4oz cooked short-shape pasta, such as penne, fusilli, farfalle

For the dressing

4 tbsp red wine vinegar

2 tbsp orange or pineapple juice

1–2 tbsp artificial sweetener

1–2 garlic cloves, peeled and crushed

½ tsp English mustard powder

To garnish

4 tbsp finely chopped parsley

1. Blanch the green beans and carrots in a large saucepan of lightly salted boiling water for 2–3 minutes. Drain, refresh with cold water, drain once more and transfer to a shallow salad bowl with the mixed beans, cherry tomatoes, spring onions and pasta.

2. To make the dressing, mix together all the ingredients, pour over the salad ingredients and toss to mix well. Season, sprinkle over the parsley and serve.

creamy chicken,
apple and celery salad

This refreshing salad of chicken, apple and celery can be used in lunchboxes or as part of a picnic.

SERVES 4

Syns per serving

Original: Free

Green: 19

Preparation time 10 minutes

6 cooked chicken breasts, cut into bite-sized chunks

4 red apples, cored and cut into bite-sized chunks

4 sticks celery, trimmed and thinly sliced

25g/1oz baby spinach leaves

6 spring onions, trimmed and thinly sliced

a bunch of chives, chopped

For the dressing

200g/7oz very low fat natural fromage frais

3 tbsp fat-free salad dressing

2 tbsp chopped gherkins

salt and freshly ground black pepper

To serve

2 hard-boiled eggs, peeled and finely chopped

chopped chives

1. Place the chicken in a large salad bowl with the apples, celery, spinach, spring onions and chives.

2. To make the dressing, mix together all the ingredients in a bowl. Pour over the salad ingredients and toss to mix well.

3. Scatter over the chopped eggs and garnish with the chives, before serving.

hawaiian chicken salad

Here spicy chicken chunks are mixed with juicy pieces of fresh fruit to create a salad taste sensation.

SERVES 4

Syns per serving
Original: Free
Green: 7½

Preparation time 10 minutes
Cooking time about 15 minutes

4 large chicken breasts, skinless and boneless

2 tbsp Cajun spice mix

juice of 1 lime

salt and freshly ground black pepper

Fry Light

For the dressing

1 red chilli, deseeded and finely chopped

6 tbsp fat-free salad dressing

For the salad

1 red pepper, deseeded and cut into 1.5cm/¾in dice

300g/11oz mango, peeled and diced

300g/11oz pineapple, peeled and diced

4 large kiwis, peeled and sliced or diced

200g/7oz red and green seedless grapes, halved

1. Place the chicken in a shallow bowl. Mix together the spice mixture with the lime juice and spread all over the chicken. Season well.

2. Preheat the grill to hot. Spray the chicken with Fry Light and grill for 6–8 minutes on each side or until cooked through. Remove and shred into bite-sized pieces.

3. Meanwhile, in a small bowl, combine the red chilli and salad dressing. Season well.

4. To serve the salad, place the pepper, mango, pineapple, kiwis and grapes in a large salad bowl. Top with the shredded chicken and, just before serving, spoon over the dressing and toss to mix well.

turf and surf salad

Here's a healthy version of a popular main course dish. And because it's Free on an Original day, you can tuck in and enjoy whenever you want!

SERVES 4

Syns per serving
Original: Free
Green: 21

Preparation time 10 minutes
Cooking time about 12 minutes

Fry Light

salt and freshly ground black pepper

800g/1lb 12oz lean sirloin steaks, all visible fat removed

200g/7oz sugar snap peas, trimmed and halved lengthways

200g/7oz cherry tomatoes, halved or quartered

1 cucumber, peeled, halved lengthways and thinly sliced

500g/1lb 2oz cooked, peeled tiger prawns

a small handful of rocket leaves

For the dressing
juice of 1 lemon

1 tsp finely grated lemon zest

1 garlic clove, peeled and crushed

1 tsp artificial sweetener

4 tbsp fat-free French-style salad dressing

1 tbsp very finely chopped chives

1. Spray a ridged griddle pan with Fry Light and place over a high heat. Season the steaks and place in the pan and cook according to your taste (2–3 minutes on each side for rare; 4 minutes on each side for medium; or 5–6 minutes on each side for well done). Remove the steaks from the pan and transfer to a plate.

2. Bring a large pan of lightly salted water to the boil and blanch the sugar snap peas for 1–2 minutes. Drain and refresh in cold water and drain again and place in a large serving bowl or platter with the cherry tomatoes, cucumber, prawns and rocket.

3. Very thinly slice the beef, saving any juices and add the slices to the salad ingredients.

4. To make the dressing, mix together all the ingredients in a small bowl. Season and pour over the salad ingredients. Toss to mix well and serve immediately.

quick tiger prawn and asparagus salad

This is an elegant salad of tiger prawns and fresh asparagus that's put together in minutes. It'll wow your dinner guests!

SERVES 4

Syns per serving
Original: Free
Green: 10½

Preparation time 5 minutes
Cooking time 1–2 minutes

800g/1lb 12oz asparagus tips

800g/1lb 12oz cooked, peeled tiger prawns

8 tbsp fat-free salad dressing

salt and freshly ground black pepper

3 tbsp finely chopped chives

1. Blanch the asparagus tips in a large pan of lightly salted boiling water for 1–2 minutes. Drain and refresh under cold running water. Drain again and transfer to a shallow salad dish with the prawns.

2. Drizzle over the salad dressing, add the seasoning and toss to mix well. Sprinkle over the chives and serve immediately or chill for 1–2 hours before serving.

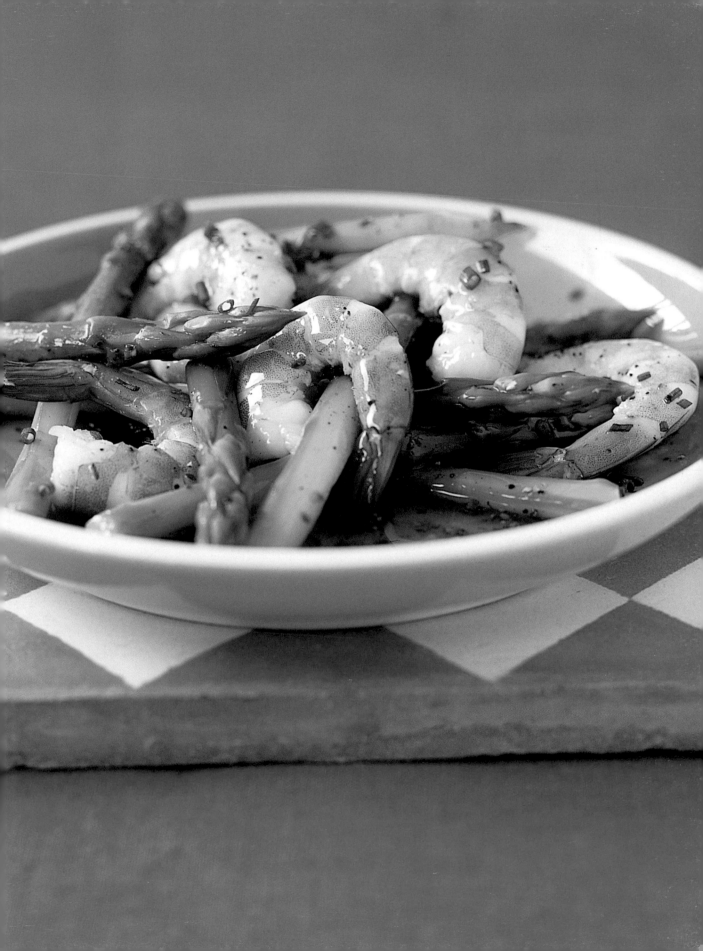

grilled calamari and rocket salad

Cooked quickly, fresh squid is both juicy and tender. Here it is flavoured with garlic, chilli and lemon, and served on a simple salad of wild rocket leaves.

SERVES 4

Syns per serving
Original: Free
Green: 5½

Preparation time 5 minutes
Cooking time 1–2 minutes

Fry Light

4 garlic cloves, peeled and finely sliced

1 red chilli, deseeded and finely chopped

600g/1lb 6oz fresh squid, cleaned and cut into thin rings or bite-sized pieces

juice of 1 lemon

salt and freshly ground black pepper

50g/2oz rocket leaves

1. Spray a large, non-stick frying pan with Fry Light. Place over a high heat and when almost smoking, add the garlic, red chilli and squid and stir-fry for 1–2 minutes or until the squid is just cooked through. (Do not overcook or it will become rubbery.)

2. Remove from the heat and add the lemon juice and seasoning to taste. Toss to mix well.

3. Divide the rocket leaves between four plates and top with the squid mixture and any of the pan juices. Serve immediately.

salmon and chive cakes
with tartar sauce

An elegant twist on a traditional comfort food, these fish cakes are also low in Syns on an Original day. They make a great lunch when served with a crisp salad.

SERVES 4 ✳

Syns per serving
Original: 1½
Green: 20

Preparation time 10 minutes plus chilling
Cooking time 12–15 minutes

For the cakes
680g/1½lb salmon fillet, skinned and roughly chopped
400g/14oz raw tiger prawns, roughly chopped
6 tbsp finely chopped chives
2 tsp finely grated lemon zest
4 spring onions, trimmed and finely chopped
2 tbsp reduced-calorie mayonnaise
Fry Light
salt and freshly ground black pepper

For the tartar sauce
300g/11oz very low fat natural fromage frais
4 tbsp capers, drained and rinsed
1 red onion, peeled and very finely diced
2 tsp finely grated lemon zest
6 tbsp finely chopped dill

1. Make the cakes by placing all the ingredients, except the Fry Light and seasoning, into a blender and processing until fairly smooth. Transfer to a bowl, add seasoning, cover and chill for 8–10 hours or overnight for the flavours to develop and the mixture to firm up.

2. Meanwhile, make the tartar sauce by mixing together all the ingredients in a bowl. Season well and chill until ready to use.

3. To cook the fish cakes, preheat the oven to 220°C/Gas 7. Divide the salmon mixture into 12 portions and form each one into a cake. Place on a non-stick parchment-lined baking sheet, spray with Fry Light and bake for 12–15 minutes until cooked and lightly browned. Serve either warm or at room temperature with the sauce.

park ride
scare
turned Phil's life around

Self-employed plumber Phil Hayes, who lives in Watford, Herts, with partner Beverley and their daughter Katherine, lost 10st 6lb with the support of Slimming World.

The proud dad gave up his favourite fat-laden chips, pasties and takeaway burgers after a carefree trip to the park almost ended in tragedy. Taking his eye off daughter Katherine – then a toddler – for just a second, he was horrified to see her heading towards a fast-spinning roundabout ride, only to discover he could not move his 26-st frame fast enough to stop her.

'Luckily the kids on the roundabout saw her coming, but I had to face facts – I was too fat to do my job properly as a dad. After a lifetime of weight problems and yo-yo dieting, it was time to take action,' says the former Slimming World Man of the Year.

He joined his brother Charles, who had already lost 3st with Slimming World, at his next group meeting. 'I didn't mind saying goodbye to all the fatty stuff I used to have, I knew my diet had to change. But I looked at all the food I could eat and thought: "No way." I remember tucking into a pile of mash that was almost the size of my head thinking I might actually put weight on,' Phil recalls.

He actually lost 9lb in his first week and within seven weeks had lost 2st. Phil says: 'I started to feel physically better from day one, so I never missed any of my fried food. Bev and I Food Optimise together and she's lost 2st herself. It's been a life-changing experience for both of us.'

The couple found Slimming World suited their lifestyle perfectly, allowing the nights out with 'the lads', roast dinners and pub lunches that Phil used to avoid for fear of embarrassment – he'd once had to sit in a restaurant aisle because he couldn't fit onto a bench.

'I thought I ate a lot before, but once I started Food Optimising I was eating more than ever and losing weight every week. At home we don't eat processed foods now, we cook from scratch. We enjoy dishes like pasta with Fry Light-cooked mushrooms and peppers and an egg, sometimes with grated cheese as a Healthy Extra. If it's my turn to cook, I might make a huge vegetable stir-fry with noodles, which is ready in five minutes, and Beverley and I like a takeaway curry – it is easy to fit into Food Optimising.'

Katherine's also happy to make Food Optimising a fun family experience. Says Phil: 'She enjoys the same food as we do with just a few differences. For example, we'll give her full-fat organic spread on her toast and full-fat rather than reduced-fat cheese. She has always enjoyed pasta, lean meat, vegetables and fruit.'

Phil has taken up squash, walking and cycling. He says: 'My GP says my blood pressure and cholesterol levels are normal and the exercise I do is good for my gout. Life is a thousand times better than it used to be!'

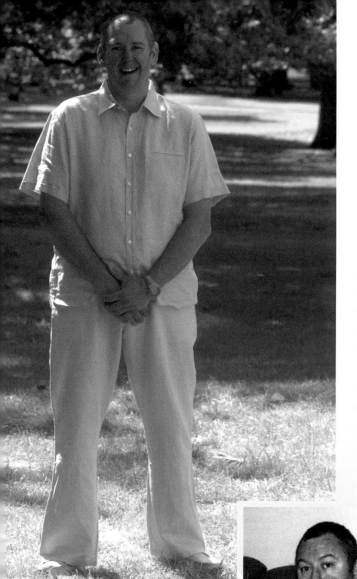

success is a
journey,
not a destination

As you travel on the road to your real self, enjoy the journey. Be fascinated, not downhearted, by the times when you slow down a little, and be proud and thrilled when you press the accelerator. Be kind and loving to yourself. And know that, at all times, you are in the driving seat. Slimming World is there to provide you with as much fuel as you need to complete the journey.

"These days, family outings are a happy experience. The three of us go out on our bikes together on a Sunday and I'm happy to pop to the park in a T-shirt and jeans and play with my daughter just like every other dad."

meat and poultry

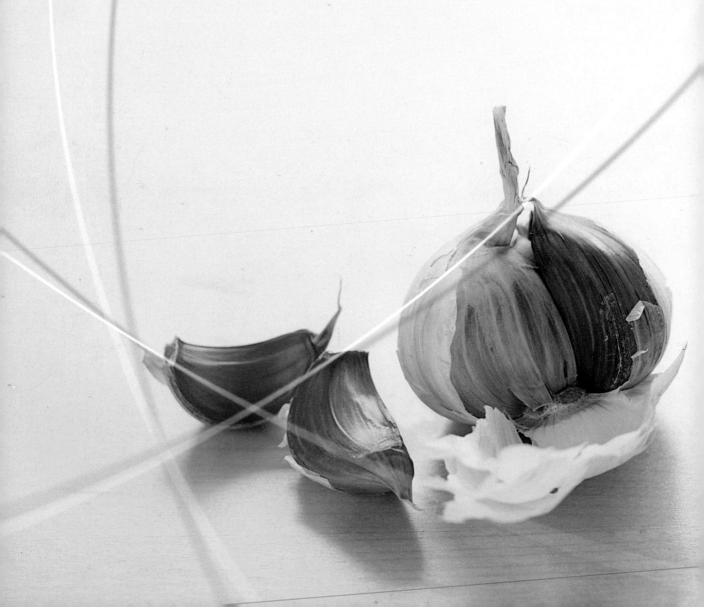

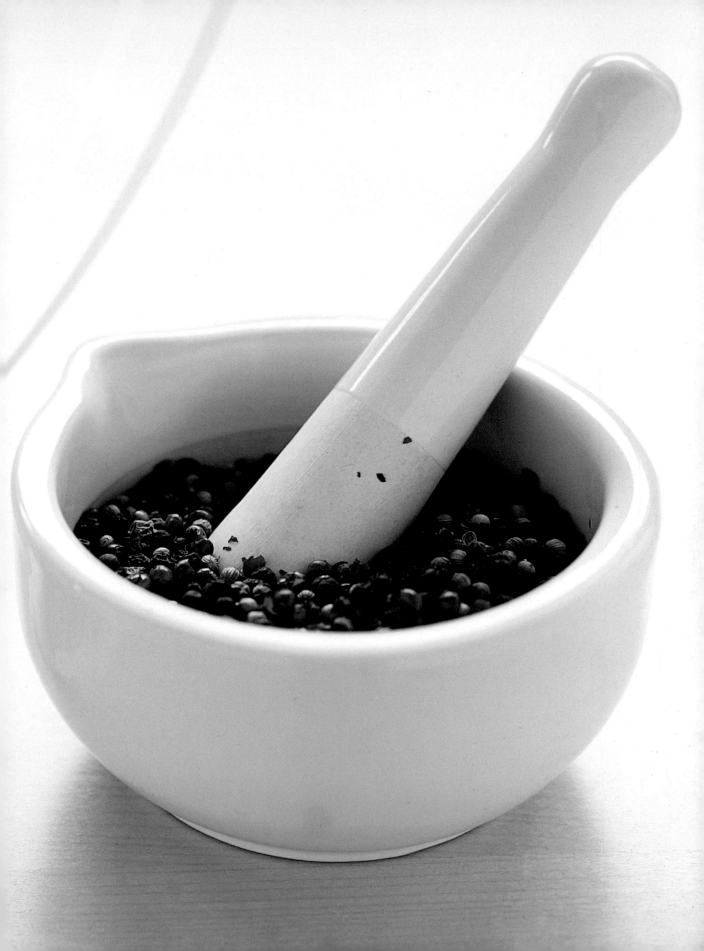

chicken
and roast vegetable 'tagliatelle'

This satisfying dish is simply made with chicken pieces and chunky vegetables threaded with ribbons of egg 'tagliatelle'.

SERVES 4

Syns per serving

With Parmesan

Original: 1

Green: 13½

Without Parmesan

Original: Free

Green: 12½

Preparation time 10 minutes

Cooking time about 15 minutes

For the sauce

300g/11oz cherry tomatoes

2 large courgettes, cut into 1.5cm/¾in dice

1 yellow pepper, deseeded and cut into 1.5cm/¾in pieces

1 tbsp chopped rosemary leaves

1 tsp peeled and chopped garlic

Fry Light

salt and freshly ground black pepper

For the 'pasta'

4 eggs

2 tbsp water

To serve

4 cooked chicken breasts, skinless and boneless

basil leaves

2 tbsp grated Parmesan cheese (optional)

1. Preheat the oven to 220°C/Gas 7. To make the sauce, place the tomatoes, courgettes and pepper in a single layer on a non-stick baking sheet. Mix together the rosemary and garlic and sprinkle over. Spray the vegetables with Fry Light and season well. Bake in the preheated oven for 12–15 minutes or until tender.

2. Meanwhile, make the 'pasta' by lightly beating the eggs in a bowl with the water. Season to taste. Place a large, non-stick frying pan over a low heat and spray with Fry Light. Pour half the egg mixture into the pan, swirling round to coat the base evenly.

3. Let cook gently for 2–3 minutes until the base is set and then carefully flip over and cook for 1 minute before turning out onto a work surface. Repeat with the remaining egg mixture. Allow to cool and then using a very sharp knife, cut the egg mixture into thin strips that resemble pasta.

4. Remove the vegetables from the oven and transfer to a large, individual shallow bowl with any pan juices. Shred the chicken into the mixture. Add the egg 'pasta' to this and toss to mix well. Garnish with basil leaves and sprinkle over grated Parmesan cheese, if using. Serve immediately.

chicken and mushroom stir-fry

Here's a quick and easy stir-fry using chicken and lots of fresh vegetables that would make a tasty light lunch or a wonderful supper.

SERVES 4 ❀

Syns per serving
Original: Free
Green: 7½

Preparation time 10 minutes
Cooking time about 20 minutes

Fry Light

3 garlic cloves, peeled and finely chopped

1 tsp peeled and finely grated ginger

8 spring onions, trimmed and cut into 1.5cm/¾in lengths

4 chicken breasts, skinned and thinly sliced

200ml/7fl oz Chicken stock made with Bovril

250g/9oz mixed mushrooms, such as shiitake, oyster

1 carrot, peeled and cut into thin matchsticks

110g/4oz mangetout

salt and freshly ground black pepper

1. Spray a large, non-stick wok or frying pan with Fry Light. Place over a medium heat and add the garlic, ginger and spring onions. Stir-fry for 2–3 minutes and then turn the heat to high.

2. Add the chicken and stir-fry for 6–8 minutes or until the chicken is lightly browned all over. Stir in the stock, mushrooms, carrot and mangetout and cook over a high heat for 6–8 minutes or until the vegetables are just tender. Season the stir-fry well and serve immediately.

chicken
and tarragon fricassee

The ultimate in comfort food, this chicken fricassee is full of flavour and so easy to prepare. What more could you want?

SERVES 4 ✱
Syns per serving
Original: Free
Green: 10½

Preparation time 10 minutes
Cooking time about 20 minutes

Fry Light

800g/1lb 12oz chicken breast, skinned and cut into bite-sized chunks

2 onions, peeled and roughly chopped

2 large carrots, peeled and cut into thick batons

1 head of garlic, separated but not peeled

400ml/14fl oz chicken stock made with Bovril

4–5 sprigs of tarragon

salt and freshly ground black pepper

200g/7oz green beans, halved

To serve
200g/7oz very low fat natural fromage frais

1. Spray a large, non-stick casserole dish with Fry Light. Place over a high heat, add the chicken pieces and cook until lightly browned on all sides.

2. Add the onion, carrots, garlic, stock and tarragon, season well and bring to the boil. Reduce the heat to medium-low, cover tightly with the lid of the casserole dish and allow to cook gently for 15 minutes. Add the green beans to the stew and cook for a further 5 minutes.

3. To serve, remove the stew from the heat, stir in the fromage frais and check the seasoning. Serve immediately in warmed shallow bowls.

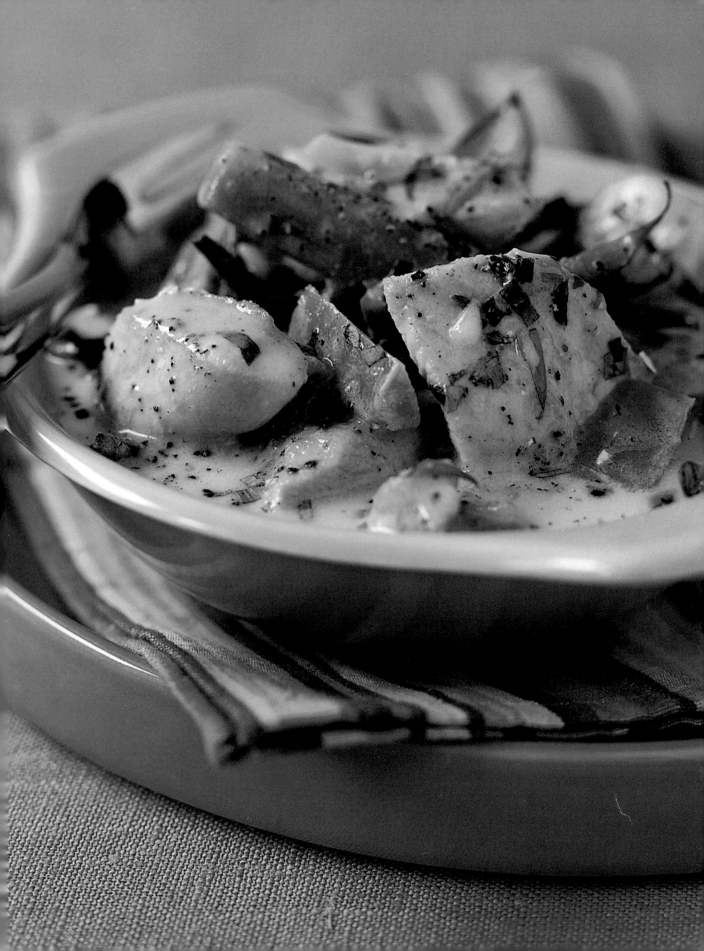

roasted citrus chicken

Citrus fruit is used to give chicken a really summery feel. Served with mixed salad leaves, here's a dish that's destined to become a regular on the menu.

SERVES 4 ❀

Syns per serving
Original: Free
Green: 10½

Preparation time 10 minutes
Cooking time about 20 minutes

800g/1lb 12oz large, skinless and boneless chicken thighs, cut into bite-sized chunks
finely grated zest of 1 lime
finely grated zest of 1 lemon
finely grated zest of ½ orange
1 tsp dried mixed herbs
salt
Fry Light

To serve
mixed salad leaves

1. Preheat the oven to 200°C/Gas 6. Place the chicken thigh chunks on a non-stick baking tray in a single layer.

2. Mix together the citrus zest and mixed herbs. Season with salt and rub this mixture onto the chicken. Spray with Fry Light and roast in the oven for 20 minutes or until just cooked through.

3. To serve, line four serving plates with mixed salad leaves and top with the roasted chicken.

cajun-style chicken drumsticks
with mint and coriander salsa

Succulent chicken drumsticks roasted in Cajun spices and accompanied with a cooling mint and coriander salsa. And so easy too!

SERVES 4 ⊛ (chicken only)

Syns per serving
Original: Free
Green: 6

Preparation time 10 minutes
Cooking time about 15 minutes

8 large chicken drumsticks, skinned

2 tbsp Cajun spice powder

juice of 1 lime

salt and freshly ground black pepper

Fry Light

For the salsa

6 tbsp finely chopped coriander leaves

4 tbsp finely chopped mint leaves

2 plum tomatoes, finely chopped

1 small red onion, peeled and finely diced

½ small cucumber, finely diced

3 tbsp fat-free vinaigrette

1. Preheat the grill to hot. Make a couple of deep cuts on the sides of each drumstick with a sharp knife and place in a non-stick roasting tin in a single layer. Mix together the Cajun spice powder and lime juice and spread onto the chicken, making sure the mixtures gets into the cuts in the flesh. Season well and spray with Fry Light.

2. Place the chicken under the grill and cook for 12–15 minutes, turning once, or until cooked through. Cover and keep warm.

3. Meanwhile, make the salsa by combining all the ingredients in a bowl. Season well and serve with the chicken.

bacon-wrapped stuffed chicken

Crisp, juicy and succulent, these chicken breasts are stuffed with Quark, garlic and herbs and wrapped in lean bacon. Great served with a plateful of steamed green vegetables.

SERVES 4 ✹

Syns per serving
Original: Free
Green: 9½

Preparation time 5 minutes
Cooking time 20–25 minutes

4 chicken breasts, skinless and boneless

4 garlic cloves, peeled and crushed

2 tbsp finely chopped fresh tarragon

2 tbsp Quark soft cheese

1 tsp finely grated lemon zest

salt and freshly ground black pepper

4 lean bacon rashers

1. Preheat the oven to 220°C/Gas 7. Make a cut down each chicken breast.

2. In a small bowl, mix the garlic, tarragon, Quark and lemon zest until well combined. Season well. Stuff each chicken with this mixture and then carefully wrap each breast with a bacon rasher.

3. Secure with a cocktail stick and cook in the oven for 20–25 minutes or until the bacon is lightly browned and the chicken is cooked through. Remove from the oven and serve immediately with steamed green vegetables.

italian-style turkey
with tomatoes, basil and rocket

Use this quick and colourful turkey stir-fry to make a delicious lunch or a light dinner.

SERVES 4 ❋
Syns per serving
Original: ½
Green: 11

Preparation time 10 minutes
Cooking time about 15 minutes

Fry Light
800g/1lb 12oz turkey breasts, skinless and boneless and cut into thin strips
2 red onions, peeled, halved and thinly sliced
2 garlic cloves, peeled and thinly sliced
400g/14oz plum tomatoes, roughly chopped
12 black olives
a large handful of basil leaves
a large handful of rocket leaves
salt and freshly ground black pepper

1. Spray a large, non-stick frying pan with Fry Light and place over a high heat. Add the turkey, red onions and garlic and stir-fry for 8–10 minutes or until the turkey is cooked through.

2. Add the tomatoes and stir-fry for 3–4 minutes and then remove from the heat. Stir in the olives, basil and rocket. Season well and serve immediately.

moroccan-style lamb

Lean racks of lamb, marinated in a spicy paste and cooked to perfection, are delicious with salad or steamed carrot and courgette ribbons.

SERVES 4 ✳
Syns per serving
Original: Free
Green: 24

Preparation time 5 minutes plus marinating
Cooking time 18–20 minutes

1 tbsp paprika

4 garlic cloves, peeled and crushed

2 tsp ground coriander

1 tsp ground cinnamon

1 tsp ground cumin

1 tsp fennel seeds

1 tbsp dried mint

1 tbsp finely chopped coriander leaves

juice of 2 lemons

1 tbsp passata

salt

4 x 680g/1½lb French trimmed racks of lamb (each with 4–5 ribs)

1. Place the paprika, garlic, ground coriander, cinnamon, cumin, fennel seeds, dried mint, coriander leaves, lemon juice and passata into a bowl and mix well until combined. Season well with salt.

2. Using a small, sharp knife, make deep cuts all over the flesh side of the lamb racks and place on a non-stick baking sheet. Spread the spice paste all over the lamb and cover and allow to marinate for 2–3 hours or overnight if time permits.

3. Preheat the oven to 220°C/Gas 7. When ready to cook, place the racks in the oven and roast for 18–20 minutes or until cooked to your liking. Remove the racks from the oven, cover with foil and allow to rest for 10 minutes. To serve, cut the racks into cutlets and serve with a fresh cucumber and tomato salad, or steamed carrot and courgette ribbons.

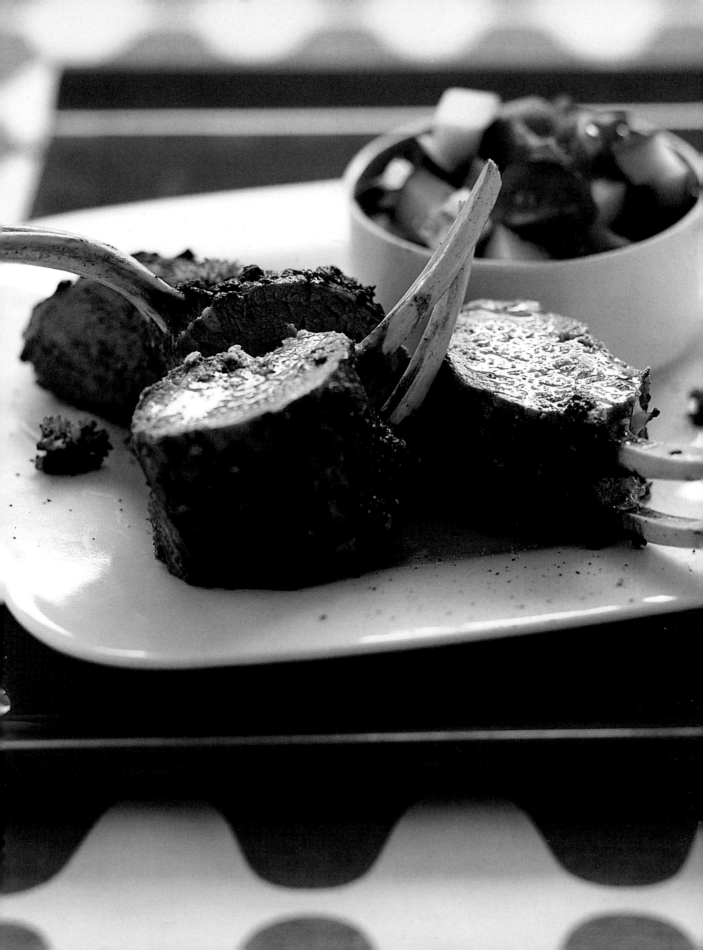

lamb and spinach curry

This wonderfully warming curry of minced lamb and fresh spinach is just perfect for colder nights.

SERVES 4 ❋

Syns per serving
Original: Free
Green: 9

Preparation time 10 minutes
Cooking time about 20 minutes

Fry Light

2 small onions, peeled, halved and thinly sliced

2 garlic cloves, peeled and crushed

1 tsp peeled and finely grated ginger

500g/1lb 2oz extra-lean minced lamb

2 tbsp medium curry powder

400g can chopped tomatoes

1 tsp artificial sweetener

150ml/¼ pint chicken stock made with Bovril

400g/14oz spinach leaves, roughly chopped

salt and freshly ground black pepper

To serve

very low fat natural yogurt

finely chopped coriander leaves

cucumber salad

1. Spray a large, non-stick frying pan with Fry Light and place over a gentle heat. Add the onions and stir-fry for 3–4 minutes until soft and lightly coloured.

2. Turn the heat to high and add the garlic, ginger, mince and curry powder and stir-fry for 5–6 minutes or until the mince is sealed and lightly browned. Add the tomatoes, sweetener and stock and bring to the boil. Reduce the heat and cook gently for 8–10 minutes.

3. Stir in the spinach, season well and cook until heated through. Remove from the heat and serve drizzled with very low fat yogurt and garnished with coriander. Serve with a simple cucumber salad.

greek-style lamb steaks
with greek salad

Seasoned lamb steaks are coupled with a Greek salad of tomato, red onion and feta cheese. They are ideal for last-minute entertaining when served with steamed vegetables.

SERVES 4 ❋ (lamb only)

Syns per serving
Original: 1½
Green: 30

Preparation time 10 minutes
Cooking time about 10 minutes

8 x 200g/7oz lean lamb steaks, all visible fat removed

1 tbsp finely chopped mint leaves

1 tbsp finely chopped oregano leaves

1 tsp ground cumin

juice of 1 lemon

salt and freshly ground black pepper

For the salad

4 plum tomatoes, roughly chopped

1 cucumber, roughly chopped

1 red onion, peeled and roughly chopped

50g/2oz half-fat feta cheese, roughly chopped

8 black olives

4 tbsp fat-free salad dressing

1. Place the lamb in a bowl. Add the mint, oregano, cumin and lemon juice. Season well and toss to mix evenly. Set aside.

2. To make the salad, place all the salad ingredients in a bowl, season well and toss to combine. Set aside.

3. Preheat the grill to high. Place the lamb on a grill rack in a single layer and grill for 4–5 minutes on each side or until cooked to your liking. Serve immediately with the Greek salad.

sweet and sour pork with cabbage

This versatile dish makes a great summer's day lunch when served with salad. Alternatively, for a warming winter main course, serve it with Free vegetables of your choice.

SERVES 4 ❅

Syns per serving
Original: 1
Green: 11½

Preparation time 10 minutes
Cooking time about 16 minutes

800g/1lb 12oz pork fillets, cut into thin strips

2 tsp Chinese five-spice powder

salt and freshly ground black pepper

Fry Light

2 tbsp soy sauce

1 tbsp runny honey

juice of ½ lemon

1 tsp Tabasco sauce

90ml/3fl oz chicken stock made with Bovril

6 spring onions, trimmed and cut into 1.5cm/¾in lengths

1 small cabbage, finely shredded

1. Place the pork in a bowl and sprinkle over the Chinese five-spice powder. Season and toss to mix well.

2. Spray a large, non-stick frying pan with Fry Light and place over a high heat. Add the pork and stir-fry for 8–10 minutes or until cooked through.

3. Add the soy sauce, honey, lemon juice, Tabasco and chicken stock and cook for 1–2 minutes.

4. Stir in the spring onions and cabbage and stir-fry for 4–5 minutes. Remove from the heat and serve immediately.

griddled pork chops
with mixed peppers

This simple dish brings together lots of contrasting flavours. The griddled pork chops and roasted peppers are a match made in heaven.

SERVES 4 ✱

Syns per serving
Original: Free
Green: 10½

Preparation time 10 minutes
Cooking time about 20 minutes

6 mixed peppers (red, green, orange, yellow)

4 lean pork chops (each approximately 200g/7oz)

4 garlic cloves, peeled and crushed

2 tbsp finely chopped rosemary leaves

2 tsp finely grated lemon zest

salt and freshly ground black pepper

Fry Light

1. Preheat the grill to hot. Place the peppers on a grill rack and grill for 12–15 minutes, turning occasionally, until the skins are charred. Remove and place in a polythene bag for 5–6 minutes.

2. While the peppers are being grilled, prepare the pork chops by removing all visible fat and place them in a shallow dish. Mix together the garlic, rosemary and lemon zest and rub into the pork. Season well and spray with Fry Light.

3. Heat a large, non-stick griddle pan over a high heat and when smoking, add the pork and cook for 4–5 minutes on each side or until cooked through.

4. Meanwhile, carefully peel the peppers, discarding the core and seeds and thickly slice them. To serve, divide the peppers between four warmed plates, season well and top each serving with a pork chop.

rosemary and garlic pork
with butternut squash mash

Lean pork steaks cooked in rosemary and garlic and accompanied by a creamy squash mash make this a quick-and-easy midweek treat.

SERVES 4 ❄

Syns per serving
Original: Free
Green: 21

Preparation time 10 minutes
Cooking time about 20 minutes

8 x 200g/7oz lean pork steaks, all visible fat removed

Fry Light

4–5 large garlic cloves, peeled and crushed into a paste

1 tbsp very finely chopped rosemary leaves

salt and freshly ground black pepper

For the mash

900g/2lb butternut squash, peeled, deseeded and cut into cubes

6–8 spring onions, trimmed and finely sliced

6–8 tbsp very low fat natural fromage frais

1. Preheat the oven to 190°C/Gas 5. Place the pork on a non-stick baking tray and spray with Fry Light. In a small bowl, mix together the garlic paste and rosemary and spread this mixture over the meat. Season well and cook in the oven for 15–20 minutes or until cooked to your liking.

2. Meanwhile, make the mash by boiling the butternut squash in a large pan of lightly salted water for 15 minutes or until tender. Drain and return to the pan. Mash until smooth and then stir in the spring onions and fromage frais. Season well.

3. Serve the pork with the mash to accompany it and any Free vegetables of your choice.

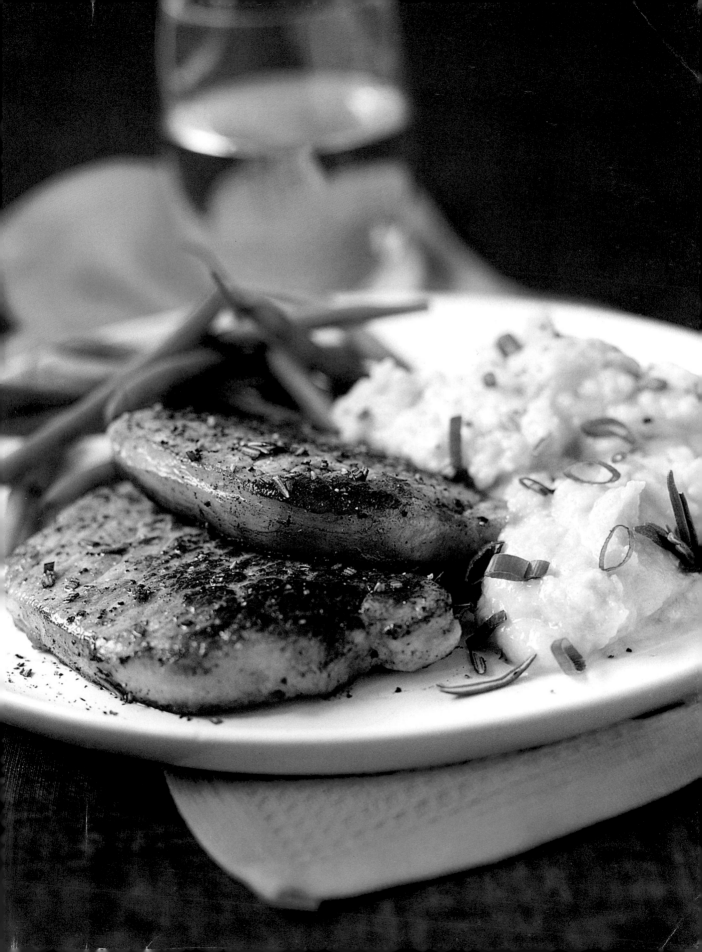

pork and mango parcels

The flavours of pork and ripe mango complement each other perfectly in this dish, making it wonderful either as an easy lunch or a light snack.

SERVES 4

Syns per serving
Original: Free
Green: 10½

Preparation time 10 minutes
Cooking time about 10 minutes

800g/1lb 12oz lean pork fillets
2 tbsp light soy sauce
2 tsp garlic granules
2 tsp ground ginger
freshly ground black pepper
Fry Light

To serve

1 iceberg lettuce, separated into 8 large leaves

1 ripe mango, peeled, stoned and finely sliced

110g/4oz cherry tomatoes, quartered

a small handful of mint leaves, chopped

1. Cut the pork fillets into thin slices or strips and place in a bowl. Mix together the soy sauce, garlic granules, ground ginger and season with the pepper. Spoon this mixture over the pork and toss to coat well.

2. Spray a large, non-stick frying pan with Fry Light and place over a high heat. Working in batches, cook the pork for 2–3 minutes on each side or until just cooked through. Remove from the pan and keep warm.

3. To serve, line a serving platter with the lettuce leaves. Toss the mango, tomatoes and mint with the pork and divide this mixture between the lettuce leaves. Roll up the leaves and eat immediately with your hands.

creamy beef
with peas and carrots

This makes a quick and warming supper on its own. Serve with lots of Free vegetables and you've transformed it into a filling main course.

SERVES 4 ⊛
Syns per serving
Original: 2
Green: 7

Preparation time 6–8 minutes
Cooking time about 22 minutes

Fry Light

1 red onion, peeled and finely chopped

2 garlic cloves, peeled and finely chopped

1 large carrot, peeled and finely diced

1 tsp peeled and finely grated ginger

1 tbsp mild curry powder

400g/14oz extra-lean minced beef

200g can chopped tomatoes

200g/7oz peas (thawed if frozen)

110g/4oz very low fat natural fromage frais

3–4 tbsp chopped coriander leaves

1. Spray a large, non-stick saucepan with Fry Light and place over a medium heat. Add the red onion, garlic, carrot, ginger and curry powder. Stir-fry for 2–3 minutes and then turn up the heat to high.

2. Add the beef, breaking it up as you do so, and stir-fry for 1–2 minutes until sealed. Add the tomatoes and bring to the boil, reduce the heat to medium, cover tightly and simmer gently for 10–15 minutes, stirring occasionally.

3. Add the peas, stir and cook for a further 2–3 minutes before removing from the heat. Stir in the fromage frais and chopped coriander before serving with lots of steamed vegetables.

mixed pepper steak
with provençal roasties

**Roasted squash, celeriac and swede – flavoured with rosemary and garlic –
add a sweetness that marries well with the juicy peppered steaks.**

SERVES 4 ❋

Syns per serving
Original: Free
Green: 14

Preparation time 10 minutes
Cooking time about 20 minutes

For the roasties

300g/11oz butternut squash,
peeled and cut into 1cm/½in
cubes

300g/11oz celeriac, peeled
and cut into 1cm/½in cubes

300g/11oz swede, peeled and
cut into 1cm/½in cubes

2 sprigs of rosemary

1 garlic bulb, cloves separated
but not peeled

Fry Light

salt and freshly ground black
pepper

For the steaks

4 tbsp mixed peppercorns

4 x 200g/7oz thick fillet steaks,
all visible fat removed

1. Preheat the oven to 220°C/Gas 7. Spread the vegetables in a
    single layer on the base of a large, non-stick roasting tin. Scatter
    over the rosemary and garlic. Spray with Fry Light and season
    well. Place in the oven and roast for 15–20 minutes or until the
    vegetables are just tender.

2. Meanwhile, prepare the steaks. Coarsely grind the peppercorns
    and pat over the steaks on both sides to coat evenly. Season
    with salt and spray each one with Fry Light.

3. Heat a large, non-stick griddle pan until smoking and add the
    steaks and cook for 3–4 minutes on each side or until cooked
    to your liking. Remove from the heat and allow to stand for 5
    minutes before serving with the roasties.

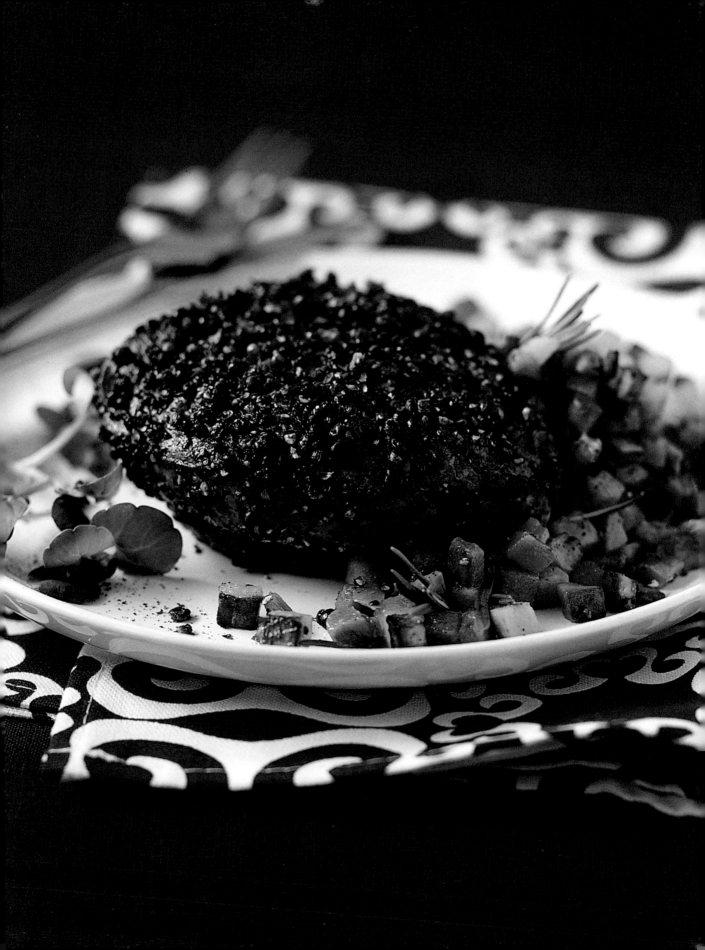

quick chilli beef

The ultimate healthy TV meal, this chilli beef is ready in minutes, which makes it perfect for those days when time is really short.

SERVES 4 ❀

Syns per serving
Original: 5½
Green: 18

Preparation time 5 minutes
Cooking time about 20 minutes

Fry Light

1 red onion, peeled and finely chopped

3 garlic cloves, peeled and finely chopped

1 tsp dried chilli flakes

1 tbsp ground cumin

1 tsp ground cinnamon

1kg/2lb 4oz extra-lean minced beef

2 x 400g cans chopped tomatoes

2 red peppers, deseeded and cut into bite-sized pieces

1 tbsp artificial sweetener

400g can red kidney beans, drained and rinsed

salt and freshly ground black pepper

To garnish
chopped coriander leaves

1. Make the chilli by spraying a medium casserole dish or saucepan with Fry Light. Heat the dish or saucepan to hot and then add the red onion, garlic, chilli flakes, cumin, cinnamon and the beef. Stir-fry for 4–5 minutes, until browned.

2. Add the tomatoes, peppers and sweetener and bring to the boil. Cook over a medium-high heat for 6–8 minutes or until the meat is tender. Add the beans, season well and cook for another 5–6 minutes. Remove from the heat and garnish with coriander before serving.

grilled duck
with fennel, green beans and red pepper

Grilled duck breasts served on a bed of stir-fried vegetables – a quick and easy summer lunch.

SERVES 4 ⊛

Syns per serving
Original: Free
Green: 14

Preparation time 10 minutes
Cooking time about 20 minutes

Fry Light

salt and freshly ground black pepper

4 x 200g/7oz skinless duck breasts

2 garlic cloves, peeled and finely chopped

2 fennel bulbs, trimmed and finely chopped

200g/7oz green beans, halved

2 red peppers, deseeded and cut into thin slivers

90ml/3fl oz chicken stock made with Bovril

1. Preheat the grill to medium-hot. Spray a grill rack with Fry Light. Season the duck breasts and grill for 6–8 minutes on each side or until cooked to your liking.

2. Meanwhile, spray a large, non-stick frying pan with Fry Light and place over a medium heat. Add the garlic, fennel, beans and peppers and stir-fry for 5–6 minutes. Add the stock and cook for another 5–6 minutes.

3. To serve, divide the vegetables between four warmed plates, slice the duck breasts and place on top of the vegetables.

picture of happiness!

Christine Stephen lives in Beckenham, Kent, with her husband Andy, and children Amy and Daniel. She joined Slimming World, weighing 16st 8lb and lost an impressive 6st 12lb in 18 months.

Every picture tells a story – in Christine Stephen's case, the transformation of a shy, overweight mum into a confident and svelte bride. After joining her local Slimming World group in West Wickham, Kent, Christine kept a unique photographic diary detailing every step of her weight-loss journey.

'Having my photo taken in the same place in the house every month, I could see that I was getting slimmer. And the more I found out about Food Optimising, the more confident I felt that I would realise my dream,' says Christine.

That dream – of a romantic wedding on an exotic beach in a beautiful fitted dress – seemed impossibly out of reach when Andy first proposed in 2003. After gaining weight with both pregnancies, Christine had found life with a toddler and demanding baby left her too exhausted to cook. She grew to size 22 and her weight climbed to more than 16st on a diet of takeaways and ready meals.

Joining Slimming World (where her two sisters were already successfully losing weight) was the turning point she needed. Right from the start, Food Optimising offered her the healthy eating plan she said she was looking for.

She and Andy gave up microwave meals, packet sauces and takeaways in favour of home-cooked meals, 'not because we couldn't have takeaways but because it just felt healthier doing our own cooking.

'From the start I enjoyed the feeling of being in control of my food, rather than the other way round. I snack all day from the fruit bowl, have a proper lunch and cook a huge pasta dish or maybe salmon with teriyaki sauce and new potatoes for supper. And every evening I sit down with a milky coffee and a Kit-Kat. I have never once felt hungry.

'I love chocolate and don't want to waste my Syns on processed food. I am actually quite a good cook and the plan got me back to basics, so now I cook from scratch, including all my sauces, and I can adapt my favourite recipes to Food Optimise. For example, I'll use balsamic vinegar instead of red wine and reduce it down to get a good flavour – family and friends can't tell the difference. I've done dinner parties for friends who have been Food Optimising without them ever knowing.'

And when Christine and Andy wed on a Barbados beach it was 'every bit as perfect as I had always dreamed. Andy was stunned when he saw me in my size 10 dress, and the day was a triumph for my sister Maria, also in a size 10 dress thanks to Slimming World.'

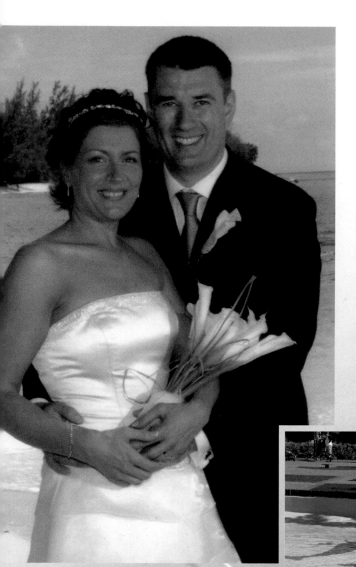

you are worth more than your weight

Never, ever forget that you are worth far more than your weight. You are a sensational human being who loves and who is loved. You are courageous and complex. You are kind and caring. You are warm and giving. You are perfectly imperfect, which makes you just perfect!

"After I had the children I was short of time and lazy and our meals were quick and easy processed food. I really piled the weight on. Three months after I joined Slimming World my husband Andy turned to me and said: 'It's great that we are eating proper food again.'"

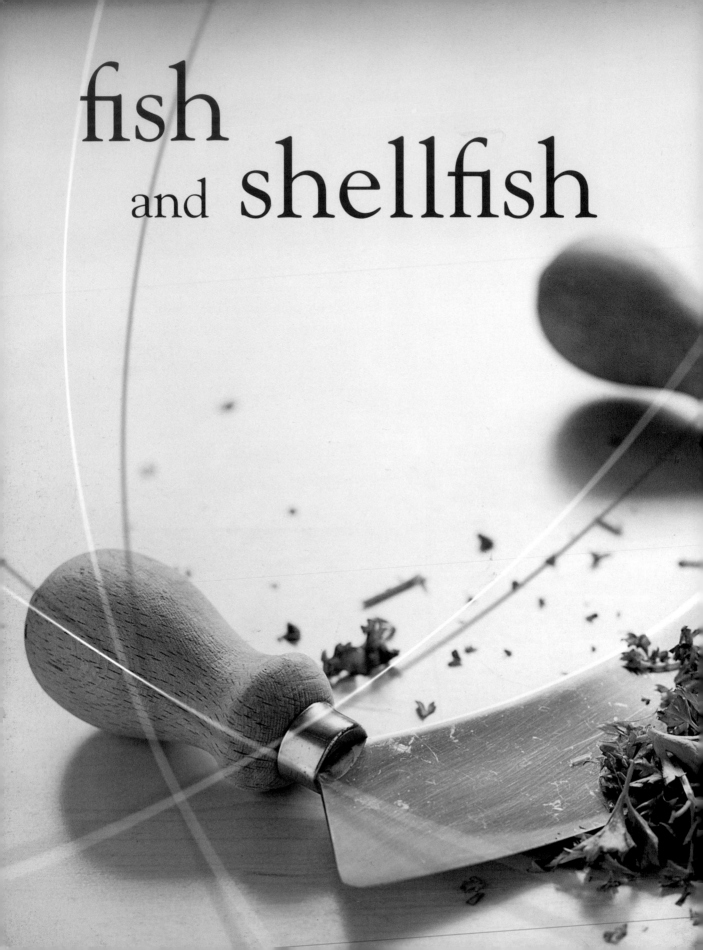

fish
and shellfish

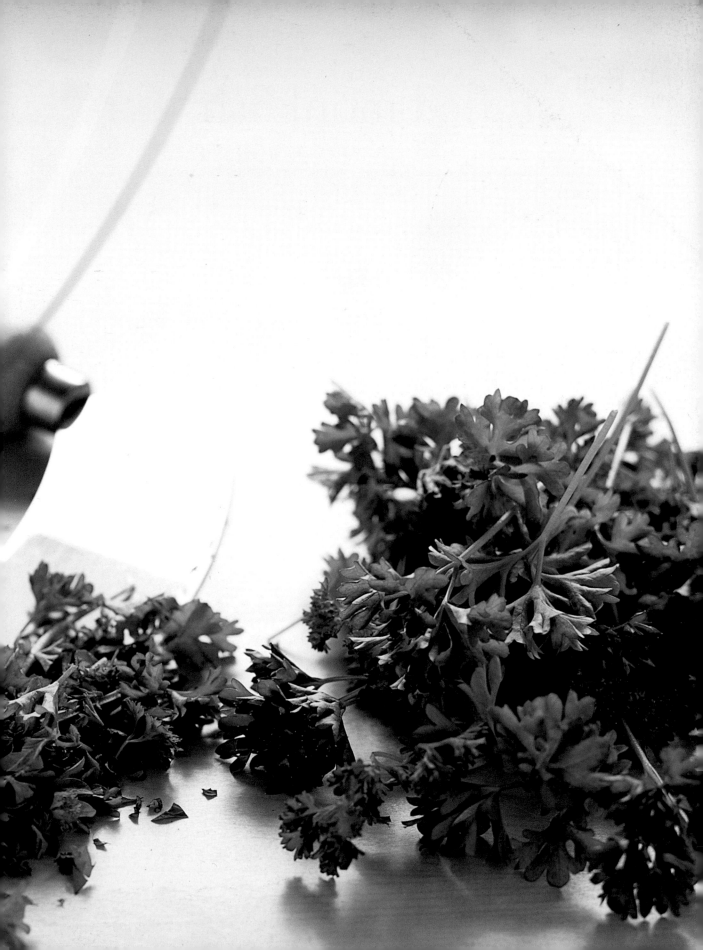

gremolata stuffed monkfish

We've used monkfish in this recipe, but any white, firm-fleshed fish would work equally well.

SERVES 4 ❋
Syns per serving
Original: Free
Green: 11

Preparation time 10 minutes
Cooking time about 10 minutes

For the gremolata
finely grated zest and juice of 1 lemon
8 tbsp finely chopped flat-leaf parsley
4 garlic cloves, peeled and finely chopped
1 tbsp Quark soft cheese
salt and freshly ground black pepper

To cook the monkfish
4 x 200g/7oz monkfish fillets
8 lean rashers of bacon, stretched with the back of a knife

1. To make the gremolata, combine all the ingredients, except the seasoning, in a bowl until well mixed. Season well.

2. Place the monkfish on a work surface and, using a sharp knife, make a deep incision about 5cm/2in long in the side of each fillet. Stuff each fillet with the gremolata and then carefully wrap two bacon rashers around each one to enclose completely. Secure with a cocktail stick.

3. Heat a large, non-stick frying pan over a high heat and, when hot, add the fish and cook for 4–5 minutes on each side or until just cooked through. Remove from the heat and allow to rest for 1–2 minutes before serving.

herb-crusted cod

Cod fillets coated in a herby crust are cooked quickly and can be served with steamed vegetables or a crisp salad.

SERVES 4 ❊

Syns per serving
Original: Free
Green: 7

Preparation time 5 minutes
Cooking time about 8 minutes

4 x 200g/7oz cod fillets, skinned

salt and freshly ground black pepper

8 tbsp finely chopped flat-leaf parsley

7 tbsp finely chopped chives

2 tsp finely grated lemon zest

1 large green chilli, deseeded and finely chopped

1 tbsp fennel seeds

1 egg white, lightly beaten

Fry Light

1. Place the cod fillets on a work surface and season well.

2. Mix together the herbs, lemon zest, chilli and fennel seeds and spread onto a large plate.

3. Dip the fish into the egg white and then into the herb mixture. Pat the mixture onto the fish to coat evenly. Spray the fish with Fry Light.

4. Heat a large, non-stick frying pan over a high heat and add the fish. Cook for 4 minutes on each side, turning them carefully with a spatula to keep the crust on the fish. Remove carefully from the frying pan and serve immediately with steamed vegetables or a crisp salad.

individual haddock and prawn gratin

Here is a great main course packed with haddock and prawns and topped with a creamy carrot and swede mash.

SERVES 4 ✱

Syns per serving
Original: Free
Green: 4½

Preparation time 10 minutes
Cooking time 15–20 minutes

For the topping
400g/14oz carrots, peeled, roughly chopped and cooked

300g/11oz swede, peeled, roughly chopped and cooked

1 egg, beaten

4 tbsp very low fat natural yogurt

salt and freshly ground black pepper

For the gratin
300g/11oz very low fat natural yogurt

150g/5oz very low fat natural fromage frais

a pinch of nutmeg

4 tbsp finely chopped dill

2 tbsp chopped parsley

6 hard-boiled eggs, shelled and cut in half

200g/7oz cooked and skinned smoked haddock fillets, flaked

200g/7oz cooked, peeled prawns

juice of ½ lemon

To serve
steamed green vegetables

1. To make the topping, mash the carrots and swede in a large bowl until smooth. Stir in the beaten egg and yogurt, season and set aside.

2. Preheat the oven to 200°C/Gas 6. Mix together the yogurt, fromage frais, nutmeg, dill and parsley. Season well.

3. In a large mixing bowl, place the hard-boiled eggs, flaked smoked haddock, prawns and lemon juice. Pour over the fromage frais mixture and toss to mix well.

4. Spoon this mixture into four individual, shallow ovenproof gratin dishes. Spoon over the topping and spread evenly. Rough up the surface with a fork. Place in the oven and bake for 15–20 minutes until the topping is lightly browned. Serve immediately with steamed green vegetables.

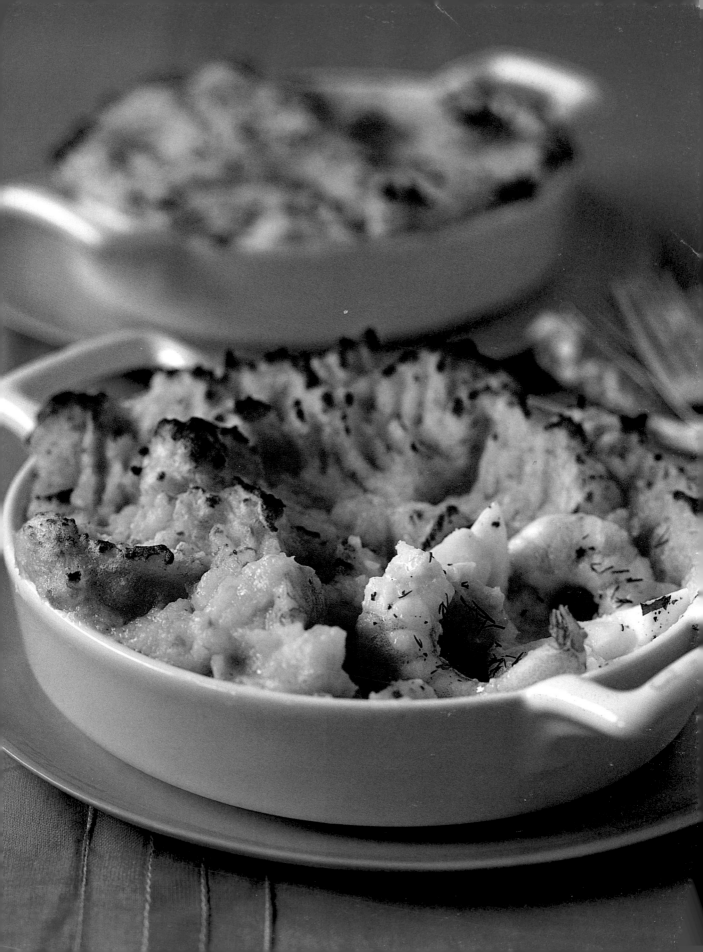

grilled mediterranean-style swordfish

Cooking the swordfish fillets quickly will help prevent them drying out. Serve on top of cooked vegetables for a quick meal, whatever the time of day.

SERVES 4

Syns per serving
Original: Free
Green: 10½

Preparation time 6–8 minutes
Cooking time about 15 minutes

Fry Light

1 small onion, peeled and finely chopped

2 garlic cloves, peeled and finely chopped

2 red peppers, deseeded and roughly chopped

1 courgette, roughly chopped

1 small aubergine, roughly chopped

400g can chopped tomatoes

1 tsp artificial sweetener

1 tsp dried mixed herbs

salt and freshly ground black pepper

4 x 200g/7oz thick swordfish steaks

To garnish
finely chopped flat-leaf parsley

1. Spray a large, non-stick frying pan with Fry Light and place over a medium heat. Add the onion and garlic and stir-fry for 2–3 minutes. Turn the heat to high and add the red pepper, courgette, aubergine, tomatoes, sweetener and mixed herbs.

2. Bring to the boil, reduce the heat, cover and allow to cook gently for 8–10 minutes or until the vegetables are just tender. Season well and remove from the heat.

3. While the vegetables are cooking, season the swordfish steaks and spray with Fry Light. Heat a non-stick frying pan or a ridged griddle pan until very hot and cook the fish for 2–3 minutes on each side. Remove and keep warm.

4. To serve, divide the vegetables between four warmed plates and top with the fish. Garnish with chopped parsley and serve the dish immediately.

zarzuela seafood pot

Syn-free on an Original day, this tasty fish soup is ideal for quick-and-easy entertaining. You could use any fish you like to ring the changes.

SERVES 4 ❋
Syns per serving
Original: Free
Green: 21

Preparation time 5–6 minutes
Cooking time 10–12 minutes

Fry Light

2 red onions, peeled and finely diced

4 garlic cloves, peeled and thinly sliced

1 tsp toasted cumin seeds

4 tomatoes, roughly chopped

1.5 litres/2½ pints chicken stock made with Bovril

1 tbsp saffron threads

1 tbsp sweet smoked paprika

1 bouquet garni (2 thyme sprigs, 2 bay leaves, 1 sprig of parsley, tied with string)

1.5kg/3½lb mixed fish (e.g. cod, halibut, red snapper, squid), cut into large pieces

salt and freshly ground black pepper

To garnish
finely chopped parsley

1. Spray a large, non-stick saucepan with Fry Light and place over a medium heat. Add the red onion, garlic and cumin seeds and stir-fry for 2–3 minutes.

2. Add the tomatoes, stock, saffron, sweet smoked paprika and bouquet garni and bring to the boil. Stir in the fish, bring back to the boil and reduce the heat and simmer gently for 5–6 minutes or until the fish is cooked through.

3. Season and divide the fish between four large, shallow, individual bowls. Strain the soup and ladle it over the fish. Garnish with the parsley and serve immediately.

tuna
and courgette stacks

Here is a juicy tuna steak topped with courgette and red pepper and finished with mozzarella cheese. It's a simple-yet-filling lunch or snack.

SERVES 4

Syns per serving
Original: 1½
Green: 15½

Preparation time 5 minutes
Cooking time about 20 minutes

4 x 200g/7oz thick tuna steaks
Fry Light
salt and freshly ground black pepper
1 large thick courgette, cut diagonally into 8 thick slices
1 red pepper, deseeded and cut into quarters
50g/2oz reduced fat mozzarella cheese, grated

To serve
a small handful of basil leaves
balsamic vinegar

1. Spray the tuna with Fry Light and season both sides. Heat a non-stick ridged griddle pan and place over a high heat. When smoking hot, add the tuna and cook for 2–3 minutes on each side and remove from the griddle pan. Cover and keep warm.

2. Wipe the griddle pan clean and place over a high heat. Lightly spray the courgette slices and peppers with Fry Light and season well. Working in batches, cook the vegetables for 3–4 minutes on each side or until just cooked through. Set aside and keep warm.

3. Preheat the grill to medium. To assemble the stacks, place the tuna steaks on a grill rack in a single layer. Top each steak with two courgette slices and a red pepper quarter. Divide the grated cheese over the top and grill for 2–3 minutes or until the cheese starts to melt. Serve immediately scattered with basil leaves and drizzled with balsamic vinegar.

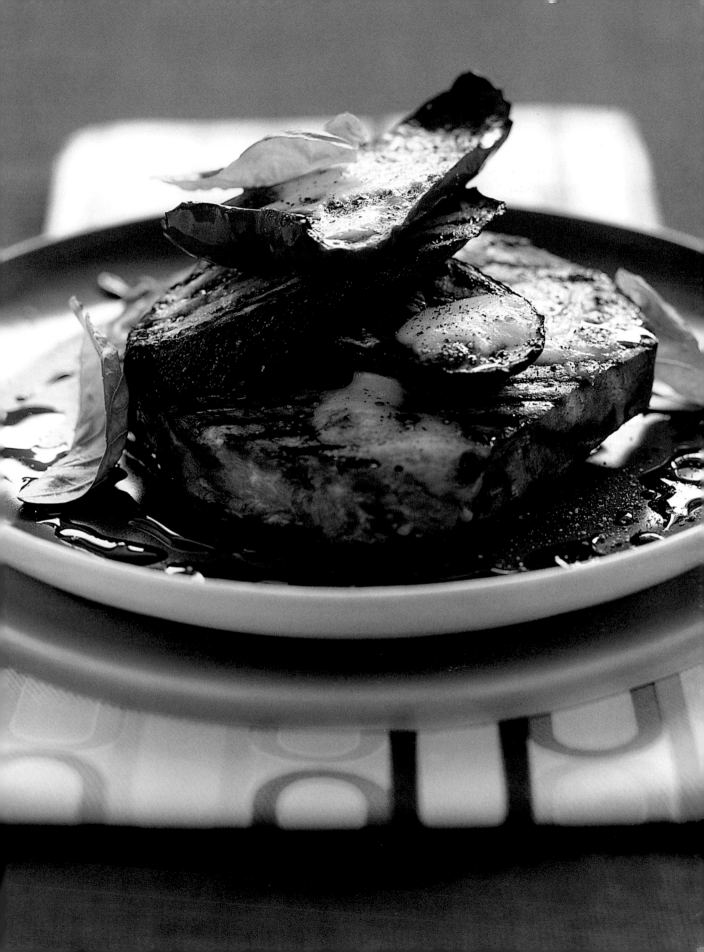

roasted halibut
with capers, shallots and peppers

Succulent halibut fillets are roasted with red peppers and shallots for an effortless main course. Simply serve with steamed greens or any Free vegetables of your choice.

SERVES 4

Syns per serving
Original: Free
Green: 13½

Preparation time 6–8 minutes
Cooking time about 20 minutes

2 red peppers, deseeded and very thinly sliced

6 shallots, trimmed, halved and thinly sliced

4 x 250g/9oz halibut fillets

salt and freshly ground black pepper

finely grated zest of 1 lime

2 tbsp small capers, drained and rinsed

2 garlic cloves, peeled and very finely diced

150ml/¼ pint chicken stock made with Bovril

To garnish
chopped parsley

1. Preheat the oven to 220°C/Gas 7. Arrange the pepper slices in a shallow, ovenproof dish that is large enough to take the fish fillets in a single layer. Scatter over the shallots and lay the fish on top. Season well.

2. Scatter the lime zest, capers and garlic over the fish and pour the stock around them.

3. Cover the dish with foil and bake in the oven for 20 minutes or until the fish is cooked through. Garnish with the chopped parsley. Serve immediately with steamed greens.

green fish curry

This is a tangy, warming fish curry that would make a lovely supper. You can use any white fish you like.

SERVES 4 ⊛
Syns per serving
Original: 1½
Green: 8½

Preparation time 10 minutes
Cooking time 15 minutes

For the curry paste

6 shallots, trimmed and finely chopped

a handful of coriander leaves, roughly chopped

1 green chilli, deseeded and roughly chopped

2 garlic cloves, peeled and chopped

1 tsp peeled and finely grated ginger

1 tbsp finely chopped lemongrass

1 tsp ground cumin

1 tsp ground coriander

For the fish curry

Fry Light

800g/1lb 12oz mixed white fish fillets, skinned and cut into bite-sized pieces

400ml/14fl oz chicken stock made with Bovril

6 tbsp low-fat coconut milk

200g/7oz green beans, trimmed and halved

1 red pepper, deseeded and thinly sliced

salt and freshly ground black pepper

To garnish

sweet basil leaves

red chilli slivers

1. To make the curry paste, place all the ingredients in a blender with 200ml/7fl oz water and process until smooth.

2. Spray a large frying pan with Fry Light and place over a high heat. Add the curry paste and stir-fry for 2–3 minutes.

3. Add the fish to the pan with the chicken stock, coconut milk, green beans and red pepper and bring to the boil. Reduce the heat to low and cook gently for 8–10 minutes or until the fish is cooked through and the vegetables are just tender. Season well and garnish with the sweet basil leaves and red chilli before serving, ladled into warm bowls.

grilled trout
with warm beetroot salsa

Trout are a wonderfully versatile fish. We've simply grilled them and accompanied them with a warm beetroot salsa. Salmon would work equally well with this recipe.

SERVES 4

Syns per serving
Original: Free
Green: 16

Preparation time 5 minutes
Cooking time 15 minutes

8 x 110g/4oz trout fillets, skinned

Fry Light

salt and freshly ground black pepper

For the warm beetroot salsa

2 tsp cumin seeds

1 tsp fennel seeds

2 tsp crushed coriander seeds

1 red chilli, deseeded and finely chopped

2 packs cooked beetroot, chopped

6 spring onions, trimmed and finely sliced

a small handful of mint leaves, chopped

a very small handful of coriander leaves, chopped

To serve

very low fat natural yogurt
lime wedges

1. Preheat the grill to hot. Place the trout fillets on a grill rack in a single layer. Spray with Fry Light and season well. Place under the grill and cook for 8–10 minutes or until the fish is cooked through. Roughly flake and set aside.

2. Meanwhile, spray a non-stick frying pan with Fry Light and place on a medium heat. Add the cumin, fennel seeds, coriander and red chilli and stir-fry for 1–2 minutes. Add the beetroot, stir and cook for 2–3 minutes until warmed through.

3. Remove from the heat, stir in the spring onions and chopped herbs and season well. Divide the beetroot salsa between four plates or bowls and top with the flaked trout. Drizzle over the yogurt and serve immediately with lime wedges to squeeze over.

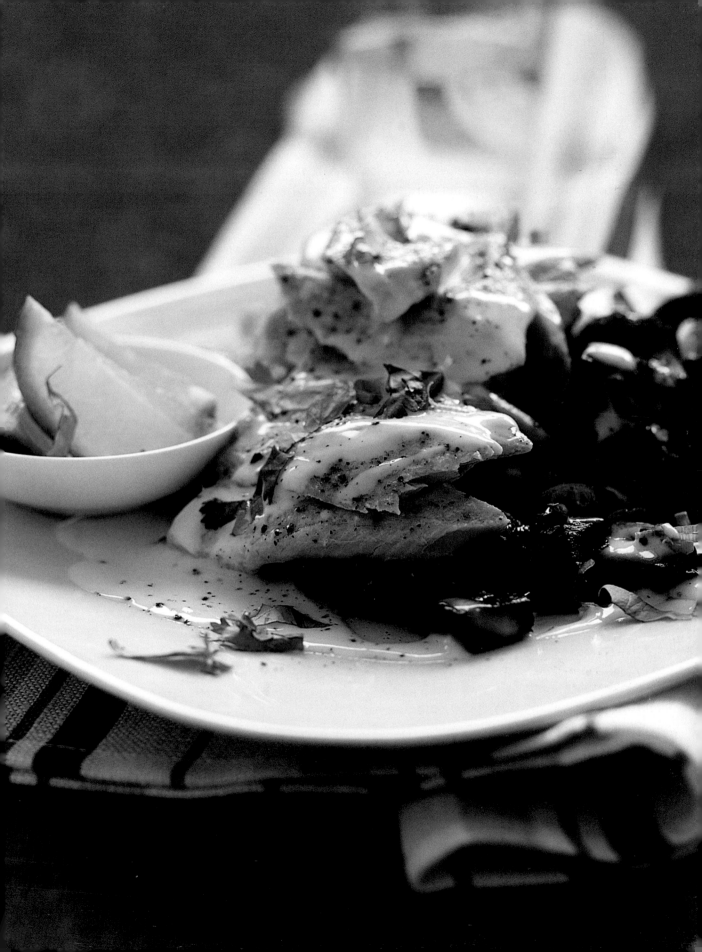

oven-baked sea bass
with bacon and cherry tomatoes

Sea bass holds its shape well when cooked. Here the fillets are simply roasted with bacon and cherry tomatoes for a great main course.

SERVES 4 ❄

Syns per serving
Original: Free
Green: 20

Preparation time 10 minutes
Cooking time 15–20 minutes

400g/14oz cherry tomatoes, halved

2 sticks celery, trimmed and finely chopped

1 small onion, peeled and finely chopped

2 tbsp lemon thyme, chopped

finely grated zest and juice of 1 lemon

4 x 300g/11oz sea bass fillets

200g/7oz lean bacon, finely chopped

salt and freshly ground black pepper

Fry Light

1. Preheat the oven to 220°C/Gas 7. Place the cherry tomatoes, celery, onion, lemon thyme and lemon zest and juice in a bowl and mix well. Spread half this mixture in the base of a non-stick roasting tin.

2. Place the sea bass fillets on top, in a single layer and spoon over the remaining mixture. Scatter over the bacon, season well and spray with Fry Light.

3. Bake in the oven for 15–20 minutes or until the fish is cooked through. Serve immediately on warmed plates.

tandoori king prawns

Juicy king prawns marinated in a tandoori paste and grilled are served with cucumber, red onion and tomato relish. What could be simpler?

SERVES 4

Syns per serving
Original: Free
Green: 9

Preparation time 15 minutes
plus marinating

Cooking time 6–8 minutes

1kg/2lb 4oz raw king prawns

2 tbsp tandoori spice powder

6 tbsp very low fat natural yogurt

juice of 1 lime

salt and freshly ground black pepper

1 cucumber, cut into 1cm/½in dice

1 red onion, peeled and cut into 1cm/½in dice

4 plum tomatoes, roughly chopped

4 tbsp finely chopped mint leaves

1 tbsp red wine vinegar

1. Peel the prawns, de-vein them and place in a bowl. Mix the tandoori spice powder, yogurt and lime juice and pour over the prawns. Season well and marinate for 10–15 minutes.

2. Meanwhile, combine the cucumber, red onion, tomatoes, mint and vinegar in a bowl. Season well and allow to stand at room temperature for 10–12 minutes.

3. Preheat the grill to medium-hot. Remove the prawns from the marinade and place on a grill rack. Cook under the grill for 6–8 minutes, turning once, or until all the prawns turn pink and are cooked through. To serve, divide the cucumber mixture between four plates and top with the tandoori prawns.

honey mustard
grilled salmon

A light lunch of honey mustard grilled salmon accompanied with courgette ribbons. Simply wonderful!

SERVES 4 ✳

Syns per serving
Original: ½
Green: 18

Preparation time 2 minutes
Cooking time 10–12 minutes

1 tsp runny honey
1 tbsp wholegrain mustard
juice of 1 lemon
1 tbsp soy sauce
4 x 200g/7oz salmon fillets, skinned

To serve
courgette ribbons
lemon wedges

1. In a small bowl, combine the honey, mustard, lemon juice and soy sauce and mix well.

2. Preheat the grill to medium-hot. Place the salmon fillets on a foil-lined grill pan and brush over the honey mixture.

3. Place the salmon under the grill and cook for 10–12 minutes or until browned and cooked through. Remove from the grill and serve immediately with steamed courgette ribbons and lemon wedges to squeeze over.

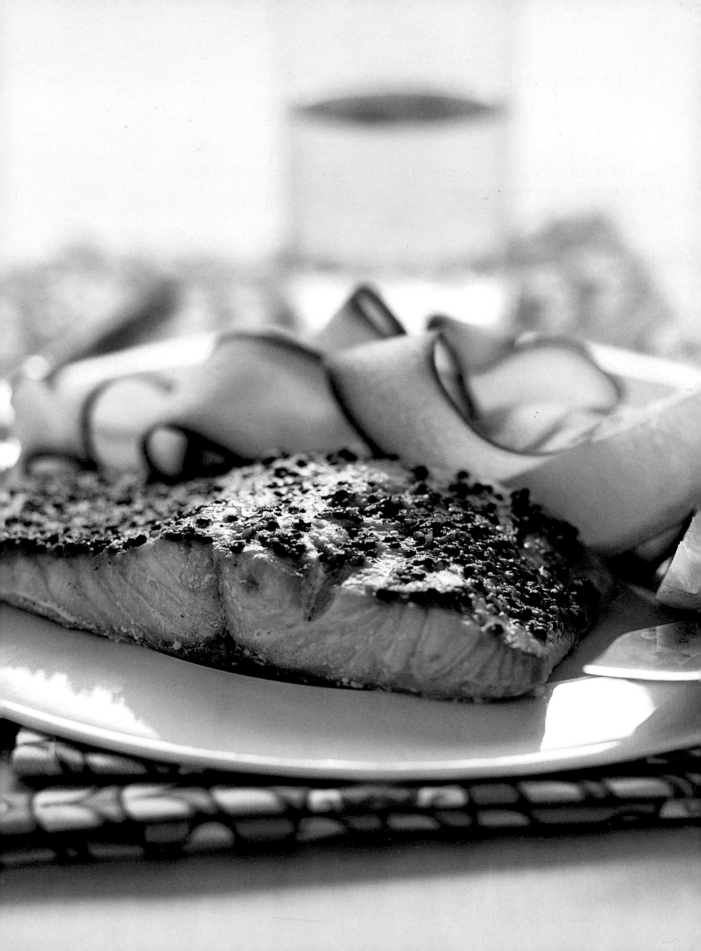

salmon and mixed pepper skewers

These salmon and mixed pepper skewers are ideal for entertaining as they can be cooked on the barbecue for an alfresco treat.

SERVES 4 ✳

Syns per serving
Original: Free
Green: 14

Preparation time 10 minutes
plus marinating
Cooking time 6–8 minutes

600g/1lb 6oz salmon fillets,
skinned and cut into bite-sized
pieces

1 yellow pepper, deseeded
and cut into 2.5cm/1in pieces

1 red pepper, deseeded and
cut into 2.5cm/1in pieces

2 red onions, peeled and cut
into quarters

2 tbsp chopped thyme leaves

1 tbsp finely chopped
rosemary leaves

2 garlic cloves, peeled and
finely chopped

finely grated zest of 1 lemon

2 tsp fennel seeds

salt and freshly ground black
pepper

Fry Light

To serve
green salad

1. Place the salmon in a shallow bowl together with the peppers and red onion. Mix well.

2. Mix together the thyme, rosemary, garlic, lemon zest and fennel seeds and scatter over the salmon mixture. Season well and toss to coat evenly. Spray the fillets with Fry Light and leave to marinate for at least 15 minutes.

3. Thread the salmon, pepper pieces and red onion quarters, alternately between eight skewers. Heat a large, non-stick griddle pan until smoking and cook for 6–8 minutes, turning once, or until the salmon is cooked through. Remove and serve immediately with a fresh green salad.

salmon, fennel and tomato one-pot

A one-pot soup of salmon, fennel and tomato that is not only very quickly created, but saves on washing up, too!

SERVES 4 ✽

Syns per serving
Original: Free
Green: 22½

Preparation time 5–6 minutes
Cooking time 10–12 minutes

Fry Light

1 leek, white parts only, finely diced

1 small fennel bulb, trimmed, cored and very finely chopped

4 garlic cloves, peeled and thinly sliced

3 tsp fennel seeds

4 tomatoes, roughly chopped

1.5 litres/2½ pints chicken stock made with Bovril

1 bouquet garni (2 thyme sprigs, 2 bay leaves, 1 sprig of parsley, tied with string)

1.5kg/3½lb salmon fillet, skinned and cut into bite-sized pieces

salt and freshly ground black pepper

cayenne pepper

To garnish
finely chopped parsley

1. Spray a large, non-stick saucepan with Fry Light and place over a medium heat. Add the leek, fennel, garlic and fennel seeds and stir-fry for 2–3 minutes.

2. Add the tomatoes, stock and bouquet garni and bring to the boil. Stir in the salmon, bring back to the boil, then reduce the heat and simmer gently for 5–6 minutes or until the salmon is cooked through. Season with the salt, pepper and cayenne pepper and divide the fish between four large, shallow bowls.

3. Strain the soup and ladle it over the fish. Garnish with the parsley and serve immediately.

mussels
with white wine and garlic

This is the classic way of serving mussels; in a white wine and garlic sauce. Fresh mussels are readily available all year round, so you can enjoy them as often as you wish.

SERVES 4

Syns per serving
Original: 1
Green: 7

Preparation time 5 minutes
Cooking time 5–6 minutes

2kg/4½lb fresh, live mussels

6 garlic cloves, peeled and finely chopped

2 bay leaves

1 tbsp crushed coriander seeds

100ml/3½fl oz dry white wine

200ml/7fl oz chicken stock made with Bovril

salt and freshly ground black pepper

To garnish
4 tbsp finely chopped flat-leaf parsley

1. Scrub and remove any 'beards' from the mussels and discard any that are open.

2. Place the mussels, garlic, bay leaves, coriander, wine and stock in a large saucepan and place over a high heat. Cover tightly and cook for 5–6 minutes, shaking the pan frequently, until the mussels have opened. Discard any that remain closed.

3. Drain the mussels, reserving any juices and divide between four warmed bowls. Spoon over the juices, garnish with the chopped parsley, season and serve immediately.

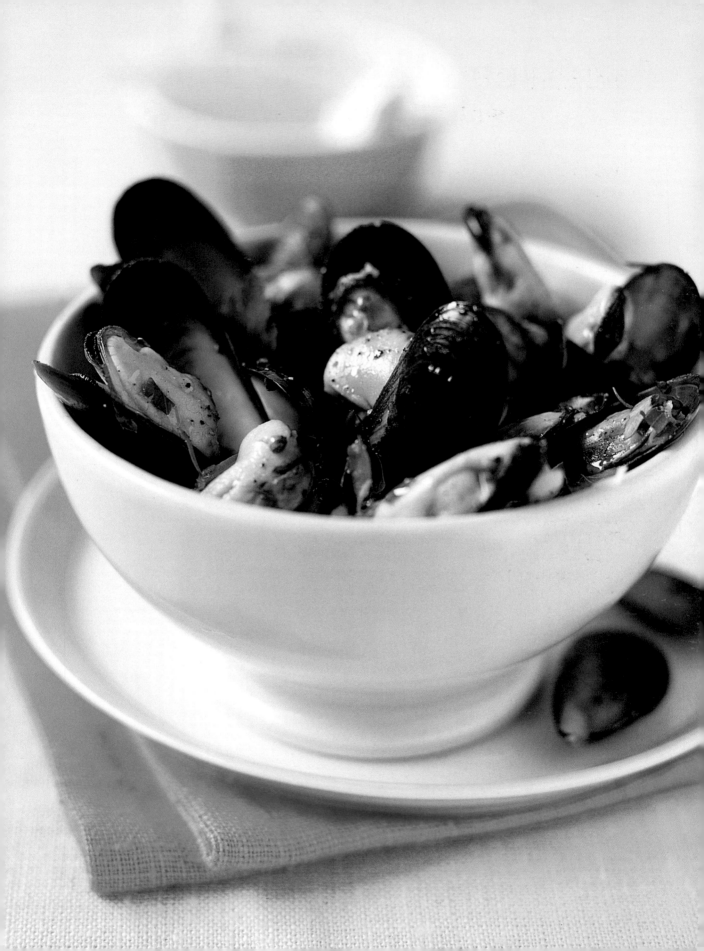

grilled lemon sole
with zesty herb sauce

Lemon sole are best cooked simply – here they are grilled and served with a zesty herb sauce.

SERVES 4 ❅
Syns per serving
Original: Free
Green: 11

Preparation time 5 minutes
Cooking time about 8 minutes

4 x 300g/11oz lemon sole, skinned

salt and freshly ground black pepper

Fry Light

For the sauce

90ml/3fl oz chicken stock made with Bovril

8 tbsp small capers, drained and rinsed

4 tbsp finely chopped flat-leaf parsley

2 tbsp finely chopped chives

finely grated zest and juice of 1 lemon

1. Preheat the grill to medium-hot. Place the fish on a work surface and season well on both sides. Spray with Fry Light and place the fish onto a foil-lined grill pan.

2. Cook the fish under the grill for 3–4 minutes on each side or until cooked through. Remove from the heat, cover and keep the fish warm.

3. While the fish is cooking, make the sauce by combining the stock, capers and herbs in a small saucepan and bring to the boil. Remove from the heat and add the lemon zest and juice. Season well and serve the fish with the sauce spooned over.

seafood stir-fry

Ready in minutes, this stir-fry is packed with all the flavours and textures of the luxury seafood.

SERVES 4 ❀
Syns per serving
Original: Free
Green: 7

Preparation time 5 minutes
Cooking time 8–10 minutes

Fry Light

6 spring onions, trimmed and cut into 1.5cm/¾in lengths

1 tsp peeled and finely grated ginger

2 garlic cloves, peeled and finely chopped

800g pack mixed cooked luxury seafood

1 red pepper, deseeded and thinly sliced

1 yellow pepper, deseeded and thinly sliced

a small handful of coriander leaves, roughly chopped

a small handful of mint leaves, roughly chopped

salt and freshly ground black pepper

To serve
steamed greens

1. Spray a large, non-stick wok or frying pan with Fry Light and place on a medium heat. Add the spring onions and stir-fry for 3–4 minutes or until softened. Add the ginger and garlic and stir-fry for 30 seconds.

2. Turn up the heat and add the mixed seafood and sliced peppers. Stir and fry for 3–4 minutes or until the peppers have softened and the food has warmed through. Remove from the heat and stir in the chopped herbs. Season well.

3. Serve the stir-fry ladled into warmed bowls accompanied with steamed greens.

roasted mackerel
with bay, lime and olives

Mackerel is a meaty fish with a distinctive full flavour. The lime in this recipe complements it perfectly.

SERVES 4 ❋
Syns per serving
Original: ½
Green: 33½

Preparation time 10 minutes
Cooking time 15–20 minutes

4 x 300g/11oz fresh mackerel, gutted and cleaned
2 tsp cumin seeds
4 tbsp chopped thyme leaves
2 limes, sliced
3 bay leaves
12 black olives
juice of 2 limes
salt and freshly ground black pepper
Fry Light

To serve
tomato salad

1. Preheat the oven to 220°C/Gas 7. Use a sharp knife to make 3–4 cuts in both sides of each fish. Combine the cumin and thyme and rub into the cuts of each fish.

2. Arrange the fish in a non-stick roasting tin and scatter over the lime slices, bay leaves and olives. Drizzle with the lime juice, season well and spray with Fry Light.

3. Place in the oven and roast for 15–20 minutes or until the fish is cooked through. Remove from the oven and serve immediately with a fresh tomato salad.

seared scallops
with herbed yogurt

A cool, creamy dressing made with fresh herbs is the perfect partner to the plump, juicy, seared scallops.

SERVES 4 ❋

Syns per serving
Original: Free
Green: 6

Preparation time 10 minutes
Cooking time about 4 minutes

For the herbed yogurt

4 tbsp finely chopped chives

4 tbsp finely chopped dill

4 tbsp finely chopped mint leaves

200g/7oz very low fat natural yogurt

salt and freshly ground black pepper

For the seared scallops

12 fresh large scallops, shelled and cleaned

juice of 1 lemon

Fry Light

To serve

110g/4oz mixed salad leaves

1. To make the herbed yogurt, mix together all the ingredients in a bowl. Season well. Cover and chill until ready to serve.

2. Place the scallops in a flat dish or plate in a single layer. Sprinkle over the lemon juice and season well. Spray each one with a little Fry Light.

3. Heat a large, non-stick frying pan until almost smoking. Add the scallops and cook for 1–2 minutes on each side (do not over cook or they will become rubbery). Remove from the heat.

4. To serve, divide the salad leaves between four plates and top with the scallops. Spoon over the chilled herbed yogurt and serve immediately.

just the job
for Gina!

Gina Hardman, who lives in Llanrhos, North Wales, with husband Roger and daughters Pippa and Gemma, lost 2st in 10 months with Slimming World.

'My weight-loss success has been pivotal for me,' reveals Gina, who gave up a full-time job in a sales office after 17-and-a-half years and switched to part-time work.

'I'd wanted something that would give me more family time but never really had the va-va-voom to go for a new job before I lost the weight. I'd got a couple of interviews lined up and then I broke my leg. I spent three-and-a-half months in plaster, unable to do anything and put on just 6lb. I went straight back to my Slimming World group the moment the plaster came off and lost it in four weeks.

'If I hadn't been so immersed in the Food Optimising eating plan, I would have really piled the weight on.'

Gina's weight started to climb after she had Pippa, when, she admits, she carried on 'eating for two'. Before long she was a large size 16. 'I was still trying to squeeze myself into clothes two sizes smaller, kidding myself I looked great. It was ridiculous, I was in complete denial and even cut out the labels so I couldn't see the size.'

Coaxed by her mum, Gina joined Slimming World, only to give up when she discovered she was pregnant again with Gemma. She says: 'I finally got a shock when I saw a photograph of myself holding Gemma on her first birthday. I looked matronly, my naturally round face had a double chin and the top I was wearing was completely unflattering. I looked a mess and at least 10 or 15 years older than my age of 37.

'I joined Slimming World again and from the start, I changed everything. Before, a typical day's eating would have been eight crispbreads thickly spread with butter for breakfast, two sausage rolls or white bread rolls with ham, cheese and mayonnaise for lunch plus a packet of crisps and a cup of soup, a mid-afternoon snack of doughnuts, and spaghetti bolognese or creamy pasta carbonara for supper. Now I plan all our meals to fit in with Food Optimising and we eat lots of fruit every day for fresh, filling desserts and snacks.

'My whole life now is so much more family focused, and Food Optimising has fitted in just perfectly. I've been on a real high.

'Now I have landed this job, which fits in brilliantly with the family, and I've never been so confident. I have loads more energy and I can chase after my girls without fear of needing oxygen. I walk a lot more now, and think nothing of a two-mile trip into our nearest town with a beach. We have so much fun together nowadays.

'I feel so enthusiastic about my new home focus and about the Food Optimising plan.'

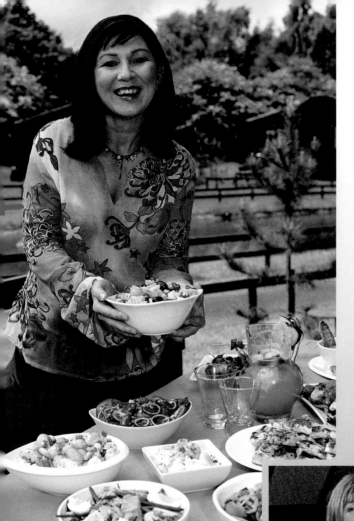

please
yourself
– it is your right

If you're slimming under pressure from someone else, the chances are you won't make it. Unless you want to do it for yourself, you'll end up resisting every change you need to make. Take a moment to think about what you want. Be utterly selfish. Discover what's important to you – just you – and you'll increase your chances of success tenfold.

"My whole life now is so much more family focused and Food Optimising just fits perfectly. We love family picnics and the fruit bowl is replenished three to four times a week – the girls are real fruitbats! And while Pippa was a bit fussy about vegetables in the past, I've introduced dishes like butternut squash soup and sweet potatoes and both girls just love them."

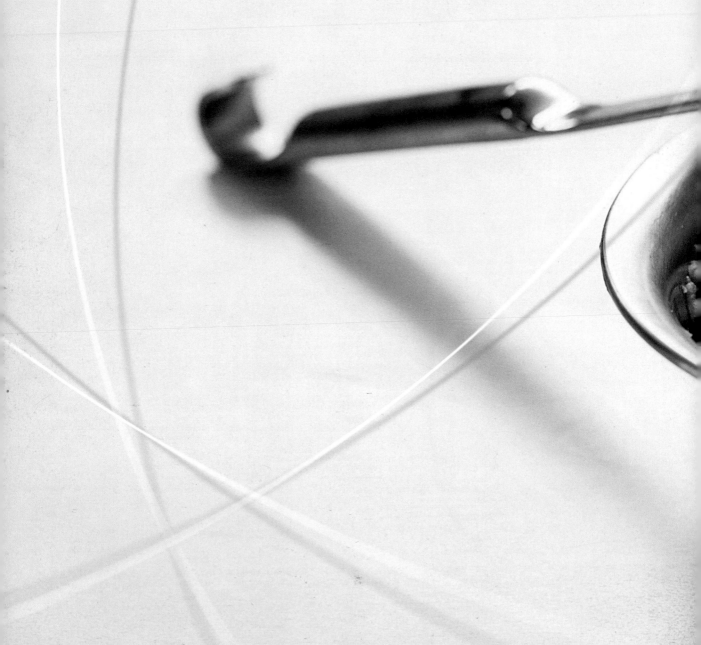

vegetables

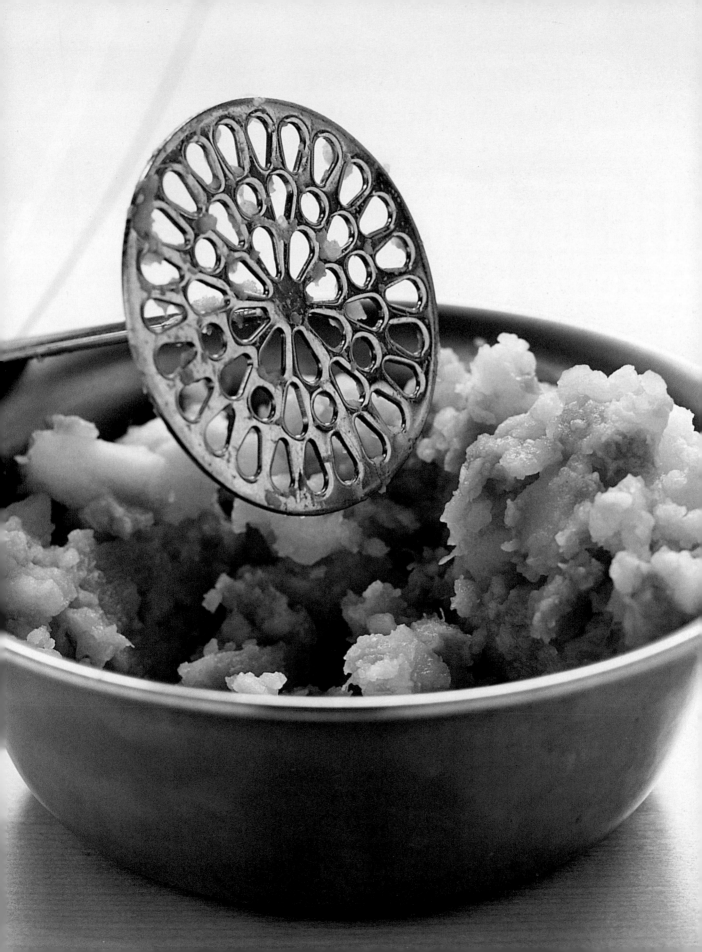

cabbage, cumin
and coconut stir-fry

Cabbage is wonderful in stir-fries. For this recipe, we've added cumin and coconut to make it extra special.

SERVES 4 Ⓥ ❅

Syns per serving
Original: 2½
Green: 2½

Preparation time 10 minutes
Cooking time 13–14 minutes

Fry Light

2 shallots, trimmed, halved and thinly sliced

2 garlic cloves, peeled and finely sliced

1 tsp peeled and finely grated ginger

2 tsp black mustard seeds

2 tsp cumin seeds

800g/1lb 12oz green cabbage, very finely shredded

50g/2oz freshly grated coconut

salt and freshly ground black pepper

1. Spray a large, non-stick wok or frying pan with Fry Light. Place over a high heat and add the shallots, garlic and ginger. Stir-fry for 2–3 minutes and then add the mustard seeds, cumin seeds and cabbage.

2. Stir-fry over a high heat for 8–10 minutes, until the cabbage has softened but still has a 'bite' to it. Remove from the heat and sprinkle over the coconut. Season to taste, toss the stir-fry to mix well and serve immediately.

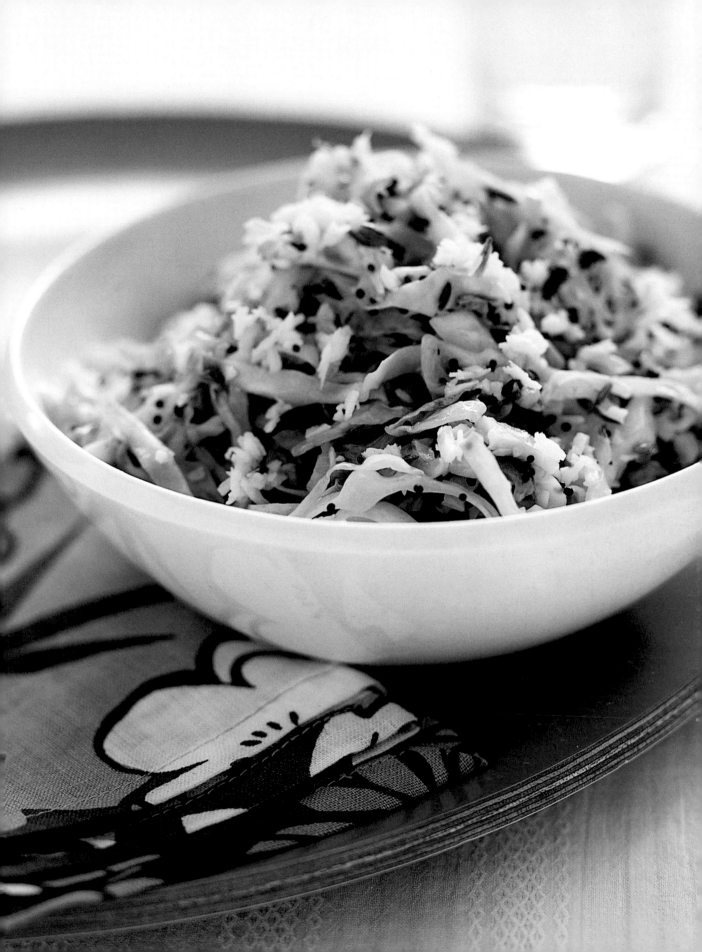

lemon roasted baby
new potatoes

Who can resist new potatoes, especially when they're roasted with lemon, garlic and herbs? Stand back for the stampede to the dining table.

SERVES 4 Ⓥ ❄

Syns per serving
Original: 9
Green: Free

Preparation time 5 minutes
Cooking time about 20–25 minutes

1kg/2lb 4oz baby new potatoes
2 lemons, thinly sliced
1 garlic bulb, cloves separated but not peeled
2 bay leaves
1 sprig of rosemary
salt and freshly ground black pepper
Fry Light

1. Preheat the oven to 220°C/Gas 7. Scrub and wash the potatoes and place in a non-stick roasting tin in a single layer.

2. Scatter over the lemon slices and garlic. Crumble over the bay leaves and rosemary and season well. Spray with Fry Light and place in the oven and roast for 20–25 minutes or until the potatoes are browned and tender. Serve immediately.

mixed vegetables
with lentils

A hearty, satisfying combination of vegetables and lentils. Simply top with a poached egg and enjoy!

SERVES 4 ⓥ ❋

Syns per serving
Original: 4
Green: Free

Preparation time 5–6 minutes
Cooking time about 15–20 minutes

110g/4oz dried puy or green lentils

Fry Light

1 red onion, peeled, halved and thinly sliced

2 garlic cloves, peeled and finely diced

300g/11oz cherry tomatoes, halved

2 sticks celery, trimmed and cut into small dice

2 carrots, peeled and cut into small dice

a large bunch of flat-leaf parsley, finely chopped

2 tbsp finely chopped mint leaves

salt and freshly ground black pepper

To serve
4 poached eggs (optional)

1. Place the lentils in a large saucepan of lightly salted water and bring to the boil. Reduce the heat and cook gently for 15–20 minutes or until the lentils are just tender. Drain and keep warm.

2. While the lentils are cooking, spray a large, non-stick frying pan with Fry Light and place over a medium heat. Add the red onion and garlic and cook, stirring, for 2–3 minutes or until softened. Add the cherry tomatoes, celery and carrots and stir-fry for 6–8 minutes or until the mixture is warmed through and the vegetables are just softened.

3. Add the lentils, parsley and mint to the vegetable mixture, season, toss to mix well and ladle into four warmed plates. Serve immediately, topped with a poached egg, if desired.

beefsteak tomato gratin

Large, juicy tomatoes filled to the brim with diced vegetables and fluffy rice. Topped with cheese and grilled, they're the ideal light lunch or make a perfect dinner party starter.

SERVES 4
Syns per serving
Original: 11½
Green: 6
Preparation time 10 minutes
Cooking time about 15–18 minutes

4 very large beefsteak tomatoes
salt and freshly ground black pepper
Fry Light
2 spring onions, trimmed and finely diced
110g/4oz French beans, cut into 1cm/½in dice
1 carrot, peeled and cut into 1cm/½in dice
1 stick celery, trimmed and finely diced
90ml/3fl oz chicken stock made with Bovril
300g/11oz cooked long grain rice
110g/4oz Gruyère or Cheddar cheese, grated

1. Slice the tops off the tomatoes and scoop out the flesh and seeds. Season the insides of the tomatoes and place cut side down onto a kitchen-paper-lined board. Set aside.

2. Spray a large, non-stick frying pan with Fry Light and place over a medium heat. Add the spring onions, French beans, carrot and celery and stir-fry for 3–4 minutes. Add the stock and bring to the boil over a high heat. Reduce the heat and stir and cook for 3–4 minutes.

3. Add the cooked rice to the pan and stir to mix well. Cook for 3–4 minutes until the mixture is piping hot. Season well and remove from the heat.

4. Preheat the grill to hot. Place the tomatoes cut side up on a grill pan and divide the rice mixture between them. Sprinkle over the cheese and place under the grill for a few minutes or until the cheese starts to melt. Serve hot or at room temperature.

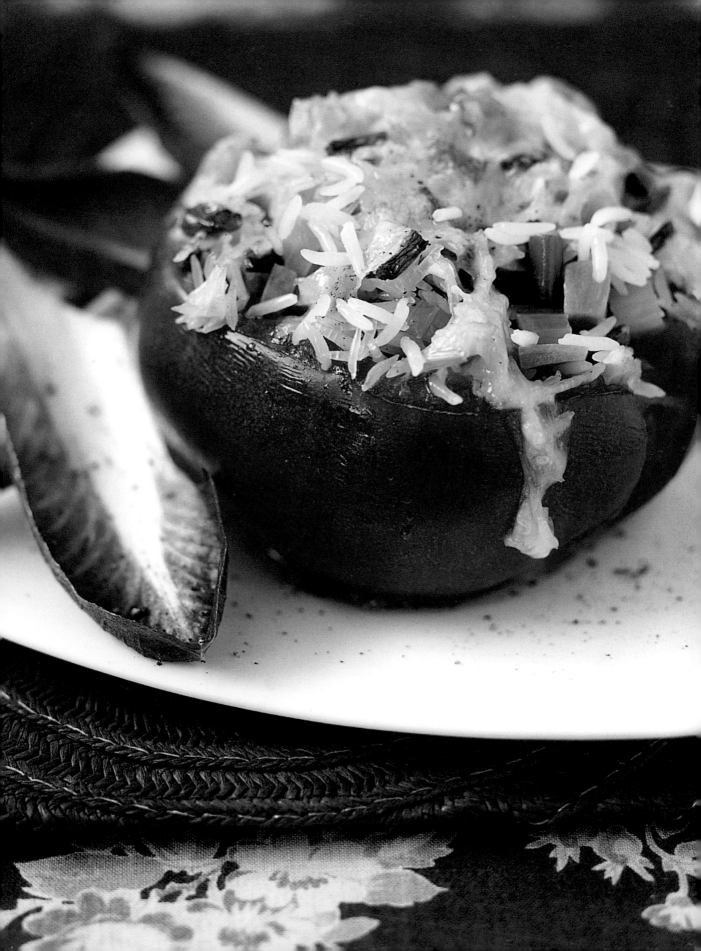

piquant stuffed peppers

These piquant stuffed peppers are wonderful for lunch or as a quick snack. The recipe is made easier by using canned red kidney beans (always a good storecupboard standby).

SERVES 4 Ⓥ

Syns per serving
Original: 10
Green: Free

Preparation time 5 minutes
Cooking time 15–20 minutes

3 large red peppers

3 large yellow peppers

4 spring onions, trimmed and finely sliced

2 garlic cloves, peeled and finely chopped

1 tsp dried red chilli flakes

400g can red kidney beans, drained and rinsed

2 tomatoes, finely chopped

250g/9oz cooked brown or white basmati rice

4 tbsp finely chopped coriander leaves

salt and freshly ground black pepper

Fry Light

1. Preheat the oven to 200°C/Gas 6. Halve the peppers lengthways, deseed and place on a non-stick baking tray, cut side up.

2. In a bowl, mix together the spring onions, garlic, chilli flakes, kidney beans, tomatoes, rice and coriander. Season well and spoon this mixture into the pepper halves.

3. Spray with Fry Light and bake in the oven for 15–20 minutes. Remove from the oven and serve with steamed vegetables or a mixed green salad.

griddled courgettes
with mint and cottage cheese

Courgettes are a really versatile member of the squash family. For this recipe we've simply griddled them and topped them with cottage cheese, mint and peppercorns.

SERVES 4 Ⓥ

Syns per serving
Original: Free
Green: Free

Preparation time 5 minutes
Cooking time about 20 minutes

4 large courgettes
Fry Light
salt and freshly ground black pepper
200g/7oz very low fat natural cottage cheese
6 tbsp finely chopped mint leaves
1 tbsp crushed pink peppercorns
finely grated zest of 1 lemon

1. Slice the courgettes lengthways into 5mm/¼in thick slices. Spray with Fry Light and season well.

2. Heat a large, non-stick griddle pan and when smoking add the courgettes (in batches) and cook for 3–4 minutes on each side. Remove and transfer to a wide, shallow platter in a single layer.

3. Spoon the cottage cheese over the courgette slices and scatter over the mint, pink peppercorns and lemon zest. Check the seasoning and serve warm or at room temperature.

roasted stuffed courgettes
with minted yogurt

This is a great vegetable dish that's substantial enough to be eaten on its own. Alternatively, it could be served as a side dish to a main course.

SERVES 4 Ⓥ

Syns per serving
Original: Free
Green: Free

Preparation time 10 minutes
Cooking time 12–15 minutes

For the courgettes
8 large courgettes
2 garlic cloves, peeled and finely chopped
6 spring onions, trimmed and finely chopped
2 tsp ground cumin
1 tsp ground coriander
1 tsp ground cinnamon
½ red pepper, peeled and finely diced
2 tomatoes, roughly chopped
salt and freshly ground black pepper
Fry Light

For the minted yogurt
200g/7oz very low fat natural yogurt
½ tsp ground ginger
¼ tsp ground cumin
¼ tsp paprika
4 tbsp very finely chopped mint leaves

To garnish
chopped coriander leaves

1. Preheat the oven to 220°C/Gas 7. Slice the courgettes in half, lengthways and scoop out the flesh, leaving a thick shell. Place the courgettes on a baking sheet, cut side up and set aside.

2. Finely dice the scooped out courgette flesh and place in a bowl with the garlic, spring onions, spices, red pepper and tomatoes. Season well and stir to mix until very well combined. Spoon this mixture into the courgette shells. Spray with Fry Light and bake in the oven for 12–15 minutes or until the courgettes are tender.

3. Meanwhile, make the minted yogurt by combining all the ingredients in a bowl. Season well and chill until ready to serve.

4. Serve the hot courgettes garnished with the coriander and the cooling minted yogurt in a bowl alongside.

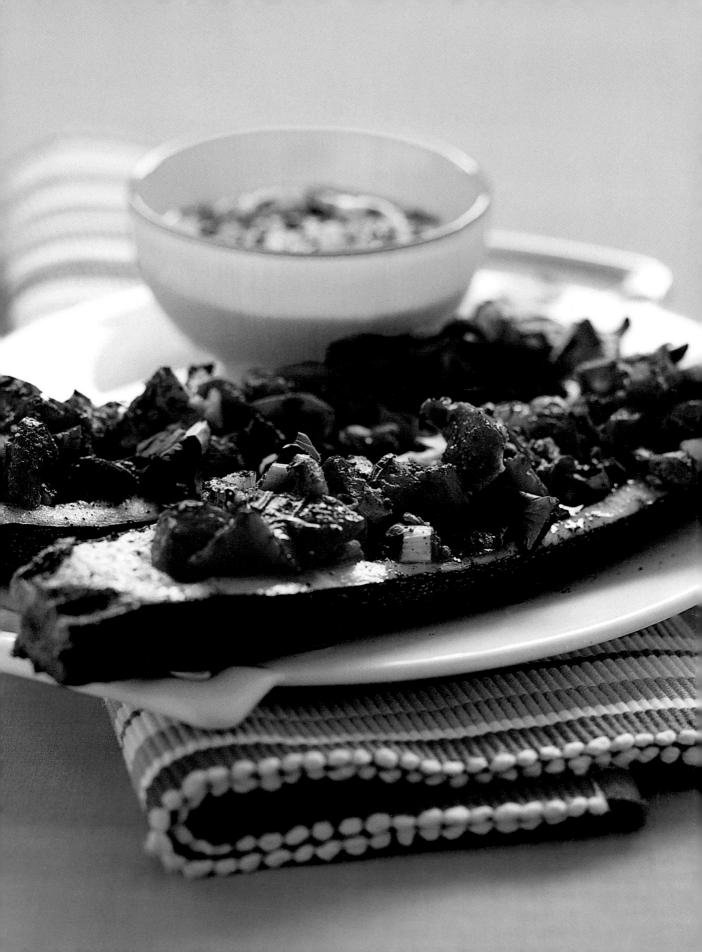

grilled balsamic asparagus

Fresh asparagus is a great accompaniment to any main course dish. Here it is drizzled with balsamic vinegar, seasoned with salt and pepper, and grilled. Delicious!

SERVES 4 Ⓥ

Syns per serving
Original: Free
Green: Free

Preparation time 5 minutes
Cooking time about 10 minutes

1kg/2lb 4oz asparagus
Fry Light
2 tbsp balsamic vinegar
salt and freshly ground black pepper

1. Trim the asparagus bases and place in a large pan of lightly salted boiling water. Cook for 4–5 minutes, drain and place on a foil-lined grill pan in a single layer.

2. Preheat the grill to hot. Spray the asparagus with Fry Light and drizzle over the balsamic vinegar. Season well and grill the asparagus for 3–4 minutes or until it is very lightly charred at the edges.

3. Remove from the grill and serve the asparagus immediately or at room temperature.

baked
spinach gnocchi

Gnocchi is the Italian word for small potato dumplings. By adding fresh spinach they are turned into a classic southern Italian dish. Sprinkle them with cheese and then bake until hot and bubbling. Bellissimo!

SERVES 4 Ⓥ ❋

Syns per serving
Original: 13
Green: 6

Preparation time 10 minutes
plus chilling
Cooking time 16–18 minutes

400g/14oz spinach leaves, washed

800g/1lb 12oz boiled potatoes

¼ tsp grated nutmeg

1 small egg, beaten

salt and freshly ground black pepper

2 x 400g cans chopped tomatoes

4 spring onions, trimmed and finely sliced

3 garlic cloves, peeled and crushed

2 tbsp finely chopped fresh basil leaves

110g/4oz Cheddar cheese, grated

To serve

green salad

1. Blanch the spinach in a large pan of boiling water for 2 minutes. Drain thoroughly and finely chop. Squeeze out all the excess moisture and place in a bowl with the boiled potatoes, nutmeg and egg. Season well and mash thoroughly until well combined. Cover and chill in the fridge overnight.

2. Preheat the oven to 190°C/Gas 5. Place the tomatoes, spring onions, garlic and basil in a saucepan and bring to the boil. Cook over a high heat for 6–8 minutes, season well and remove from the heat. Spoon this mixture over the base of a medium, shallow ovenproof dish.

3. Make the gnocchi by taking walnut-sized pieces of the potato mixture and shaping them into balls or cylindrical shapes. Place them in a single layer over the tomato mixture. Sprinkle over the grated cheese and bake in the oven for 10 minutes until hot and bubbling. Serve immediately with a crisp green salad.

sautéed mushrooms
with red onion, garlic and parsley

The harmonious combination of mushrooms, garlic, red onion and flat-leaf parsley makes this a great accompaniment to rice or noodles. It would be wonderful with chicken or fish on an Original day, too!

SERVES 4 Ⓥ

Syns per serving
Original: Free
Green: Free

Preparation time 6–8 minutes
Cooking time 10–12 minutes

12 large portobello
mushrooms

Fry Light

4 garlic cloves, peeled and
thinly sliced

1 red onion, peeled and finely
diced

salt and freshly ground black
pepper

a large handful of flat-leaf
parsley, roughly chopped

1. Wipe the mushrooms and cut into 1cm/½in-thick slices.

2. Spray a large non-stick frying pan with Fry Light and place over a high heat. Add the garlic, red onion and mushrooms, season well and stir and cook over a high heat for 10–12 minutes, until all the liquid that was released by the mushrooms is absorbed.

3. Remove from the heat, stir in the chopped parsley and serve immediately with some steamed brown rice or noodles.

creamy dijon mustard
cauliflower cheese

Traditional cauliflower cheese is taken a step further with the addition of spring onions and Dijon mustard. A great Sunday lunch partner.

SERVES 4 ⓥ ❄

Syns per serving
Original: 4½
Green: 4½

Preparation time 10 minutes
Cooking time 12–15 minutes

800g/1lb 12oz cauliflower florets

6 spring onions, trimmed and finely sliced

400g/14oz Total 0% Greek natural yogurt

2 tsp Dijon mustard

110g/4oz reduced fat Cheddar cheese, grated

salt and freshly ground black pepper

1. Boil the cauliflower florets in a large saucepan of lightly salted water for 6–8 minutes or until just tender. Drain and transfer to a shallow ovenproof dish. Sprinkle over the spring onions.

2. Mix together the yogurt, mustard and cheese. Season well and pour this mixture over the cauliflower to cover.

3. Preheat the grill to medium-hot. Place the dish under the grill for 5–6 minutes or until lightly golden and bubbling. Serve immediately with steamed green vegetables or a tomato salad.

moroccan-style
carrots

Here's a spicy way to liven up carrots. They would be wonderful served with a meat or fish dish.

SERVES 4 Ⓥ ❋
Syns per serving
Original: Free
Green: Free

Preparation time 5 minutes
Cooking time about 25 minutes

Fry Light

1 red onion, peeled, halved and thinly sliced

1 tsp ground cumin

1 tsp ground cinnamon

1 tsp cayenne pepper

¼ tsp ground cardamom seeds

1kg/2lb 4oz carrots, peeled and cut into thick batons

250ml/9fl oz boiling water or vegetable stock made with Vecon

4 tbsp finely chopped coriander leaves

salt and freshly ground black pepper

1. Spray a large, non-stick saucepan with Fry Light and place over a medium heat. Add the red onion and stir-fry for 2–3 minutes.

2. Stir in the cumin, cinnamon, cayenne pepper and cardamom and stir-fry for 30–40 seconds. Add the carrots and stir for 1–2 minutes over a high heat.

3. Pour in the water or stock, bring to the boil, cover tightly, reduce the heat to low and simmer gently for 15–20 minutes or until most of the liquid is absorbed and the carrots are tender. Remove from the heat and sprinkle over the coriander. Season well and serve immediately.

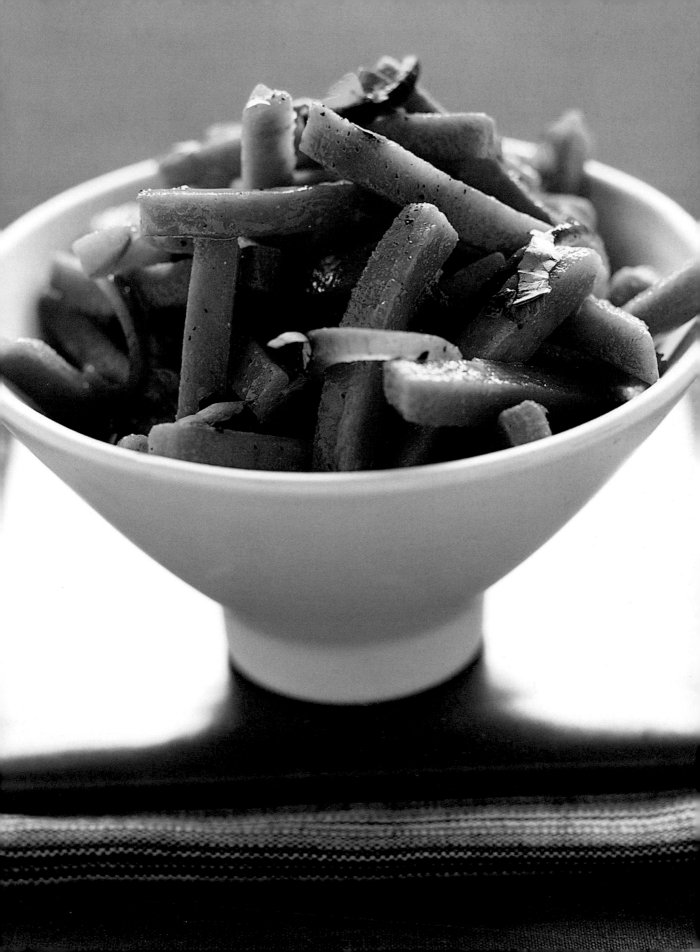

minted
mushy peas

These are an absolute must for Bonfire Night and after you've tasted them, you'll want them on your menu more than once a year.

SERVES 4 Ⓥ ❄

Syns per serving
Original: 9
Green: Free

Preparation time 5 minutes
Cooking time about 6 minutes

1kg/2lb 4oz fresh or frozen peas

6 spring onions, finely chopped

200g/7oz very low fat natural fromage frais

a small handful of mint leaves, chopped

salt and freshly ground black pepper

1. Bring a large pan of lightly salted water to the boil. Add the peas and bring back to the boil. Reduce the heat and simmer for 4–5 minutes or until the peas are cooked and drain thoroughly.

2. Place the peas in a food processor with the spring onions, fromage frais and mint. Season well and process until the mixture is fairly smooth.

3. Serve the peas immediately with boiled potatoes and carrots.

herbed
vegetable quiche

Quiche is great for lunchboxes and picnics and this recipe is no exception. It has the added bonus of being low in Syns on a Green day, too!

SERVES 4 Ⓥ ❄

Syns per serving
Original: 4½
Green: 3½

Preparation time 10 minutes
Cooking time 20–25 minutes

Fry Light

6 spring onions, trimmed and finely sliced

2 garlic cloves, peeled and finely chopped

110g/4oz cooked carrots, cut into 1cm/½in dice

110g/4oz cooked potatoes, cut into 1cm/½in dice

200g/7oz roasted red pepper, cut into 1cm/½in dice

110g/4oz feta cheese

4 eggs

6 tbsp finely chopped mixed herbs, such as parsley, dill, tarragon and chives

salt and freshly ground black pepper

1. Preheat the oven to 220°C/Gas 7. Lightly spray a 20cm/8in square ovenproof dish with Fry Light.

2. Mix together the spring onions, garlic, carrots, potatoes, red pepper and feta cheese and spoon into the prepared dish in an even layer.

3. Whisk the eggs with the chopped herbs, season well and pour over the vegetable mixture. Place in the oven and bake for 20–25 minutes or until golden and just set. Remove from the oven and allow to stand for 10–12 minutes before cutting into squares and eating.

spinach and chickpea one-pot

A comforting spinach and chickpea 'soup' that's perfect for wintry weather. Just add a roaring open fire – bliss!

SERVES 4 Ⓥ ✳

Syns per serving
Original: 10½
Green: Free

Preparation time 10 minutes
Cooking time about 10 minutes

Fry Light

2 red onions, peeled, halved and thinly sliced

2 garlic cloves, peeled and crushed

2 tsp cumin seeds

1 tsp peeled and finely grated ginger

1 tbsp mild curry powder

300ml/½ pint boiling water or vegetable stock made with Vecon

4 plum tomatoes, roughly chopped

2 x 400g cans chickpeas, drained and rinsed

250g/9oz baby spinach leaves

salt and freshly ground black pepper

1. Lightly spray a large, non-stick wok or frying pan with Fry Light and place over a medium heat. Add the red onions and stir-fry for 5 minutes. Add the garlic, cumin seeds, ginger and curry powder and stir-fry for 1–2 minutes.

2. Add the water or stock and tomatoes and bring to the boil. Stir in the chickpeas and spinach, bring back to the boil and cook for 2–3 minutes or until the chickpeas are heated through and the spinach has wilted. Season well and serve immediately.

tofu and vegetable burgers
with dilled cucumber relish

These tofu and vegetable burgers are a great vegetarian alternative to meat and fish when barbecuing, and the tangy relish is the perfect partner.

SERVES 4 Ⓥ ❋

Syns per serving
Original: 6½
Green: Free

Preparation time 10 minutes
plus chilling

Cooking time about 12–16
minutes

For the burgers

500g/1lb 2oz mashed potato,
chilled

200g/7oz peas (fresh or
thawed frozen)

2 spring onions, trimmed and
roughly chopped

4 tbsp finely chopped flat-leaf
parsley

2 tbsp finely chopped chives

300g/11oz firm tofu

1 small egg

salt and freshly ground black
pepper

Fry Light

For the relish

1 cucumber, halved and thinly
sliced

4 tbsp finely chopped dill

2 tbsp raspberry vinegar

To serve

mixed salad leaves

1. To make the burgers, combine all the ingredients, except the seasoning and Fry Light, in a food processor and process until smooth. Season well and transfer to a bowl, cover and chill in the fridge for 8–10 hours or overnight to firm up the mixture.

2. To make the relish, combine all the ingredients in a bowl. Season well and set aside.

3. When ready to eat, preheat the grill to medium-hot. Divide the burger mixture into 8–12 portions and form each one into a ball. Flatten each one slightly and place on a grill rack. Spray with Fry Light and grill for 6–8 minutes on each side until lightly golden. Serve immediately with the relish and crisp mixed salad leaves.

oven-roasted tomatoes
with thyme

Just imagine some fresh juicy tomatoes, seasoned and roasted in the oven until they've collapsed slightly. They can be eaten at room temperature – if you can resist them that long!

SERVES 4 (V) (✲)

Syns per serving
Original: 1½
Green: 1½

Preparation time 5 minutes
Cooking time 15–20 minutes

1kg/2lb 4oz midi vine plum tomatoes
Fry Light
1 tbsp olive oil
4 garlic cloves, peeled and finely chopped
salt and freshly ground black pepper

To garnish
a small handful of thyme leaves

1. Preheat the oven to 220°C/Gas 7. Place the tomatoes on a non-stick baking tray in a single layer.

2. Spray with Fry Light and drizzle over the olive oil. Scatter over the garlic and season well.

3. Place in the oven and roast for 15–20 minutes until tender. Remove from the oven and sprinkle over the thyme. Eat warm or at room temperature.

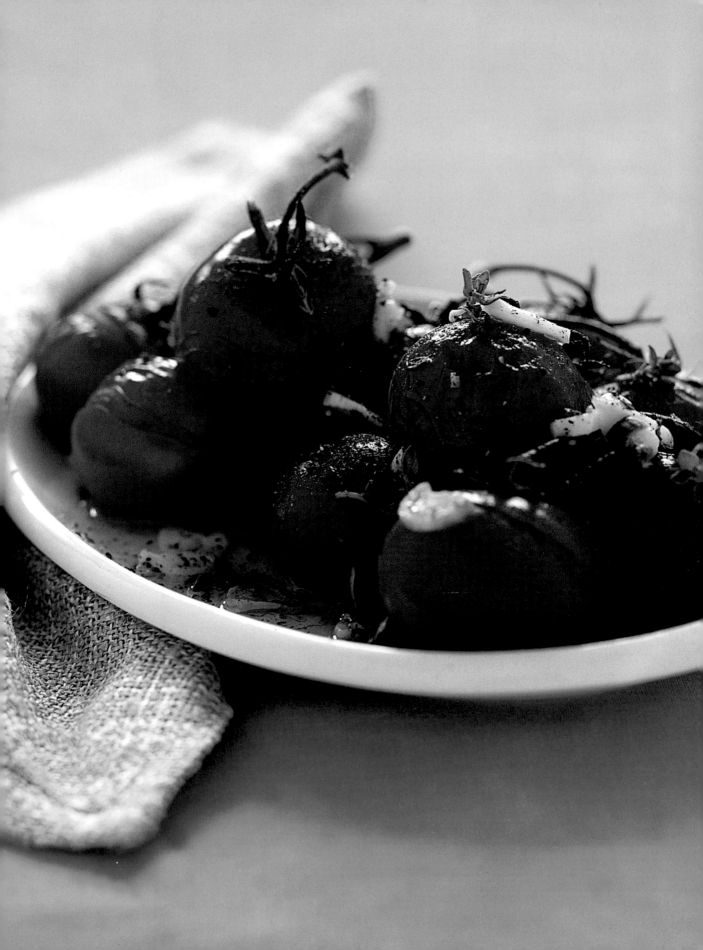

dramatic difference for Sophie

Teenager Sophie Jenkins lives in Rumney, Cardiff, with her dad Wayne, stepmother Tina, sister Victoria, stepbrother Gareth and stepsister Hayley. Mum Teresa lives close by.

Drama student Sophie Jenkins became something of a school 'health guru' after transforming her lifestyle and her self-confidence with the help of Slimming World.

'I spread the healthy eating message to my friends,' says Sophie. 'Most of the time they don't believe how much I eat. Typically, I enjoy breakfast of bran flakes and chopped-up fruit, which I eat like fruit crumble because I don't drink milk. Dinner is usually a Free meal, such as a jacket potato with beans on a Green day or ham salad on an Original day, and then an evening meal of rice with chilli, spaghetti bolognese or a stir-fry.'

Sophie began gaining weight at 11 years old and found her confidence dented by the sight of unflattering holiday photographs. She joined a Slimming World group with her aunt and, initially nervous at being the youngest member, at 15, she soon found it warm and comforting.

'It was a new experience for Tracey, my Consultant, too, as she'd never had anyone my age in her group. I had to have a note from my doctor before I could start Food Optimising, and I was allowed a few more Healthy Extras than normal.'

Sophie was delighted to discover that Slimming World's healthy eating advice allowed her lots of freedom to enjoy her food – and she lost more than a stone-and-a-half! 'I'm a big chocoholic and I love my food. With Food Optimising I can fill up on all the Free Foods and not have to cut down my portion sizes.

'My favourite Green choice meal is pasta with tuna and sweetcorn and cheese melted on the top. Most of my meals are Syn-free so I can save my Syns for chocolate. I also love cherry-flavour Müllerlight yogurts. I freeze them so it's just like eating ice cream!'

'And while I wasn't terribly interested in exercise when I was younger, I really enjoy it now. I used to hate walking to college or standing up on buses. I used to feel everyone was looking at me and I was forever fiddling with my clothes, wondering what I looked like. I never used to wear high heels because I thought they'd break. Now I walk to college every day and do aerobics with my mum three times a week. I love the way it makes me feel so good afterwards. Then, of course, there's all the dancing around the stage at rehearsals!'

After maintaining her weight at a healthy 11st for more than a year, Sophie is confident she can carry on Food Optimising when she embarks on an exciting teaching placement in Fiji. She'll then take up a place at Aberystwyth University where she is to study drama.

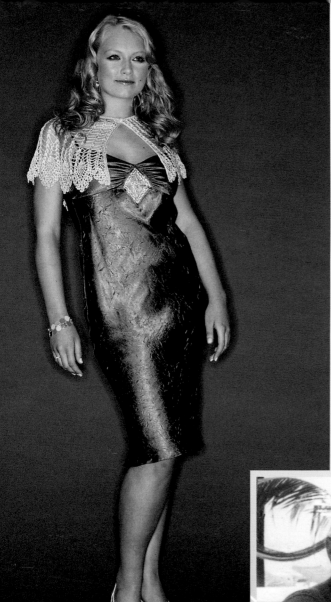

live the dream

Believe in the dream. And then live it. No matter how busy your day, take some time to close your eyes and picture your dream in all its full-colour glory. See it happening, feel the feelings that are yours to claim on realising your dream. Don't let it fade. Keep your dream alive by feeding it, nurturing it and visiting it every day.

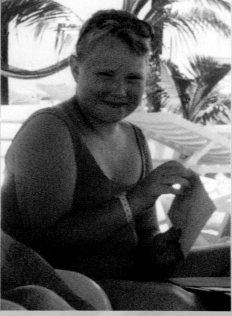

"Cooking at home wasn't a problem because my dad and sister joined Slimming World as well, so we all ate the same things."

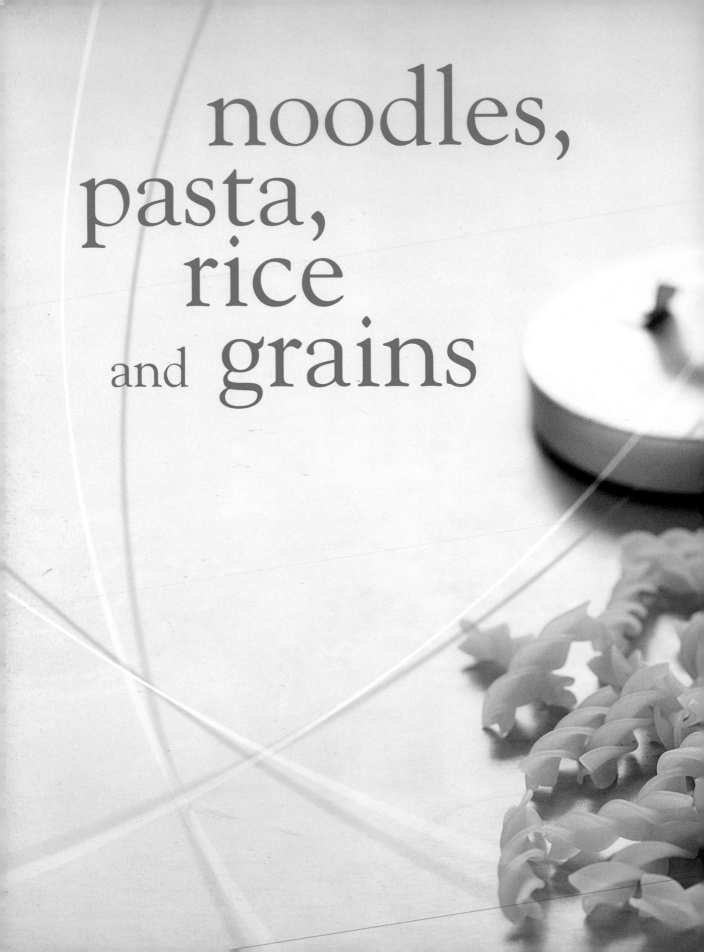

noodles, pasta, rice and grains

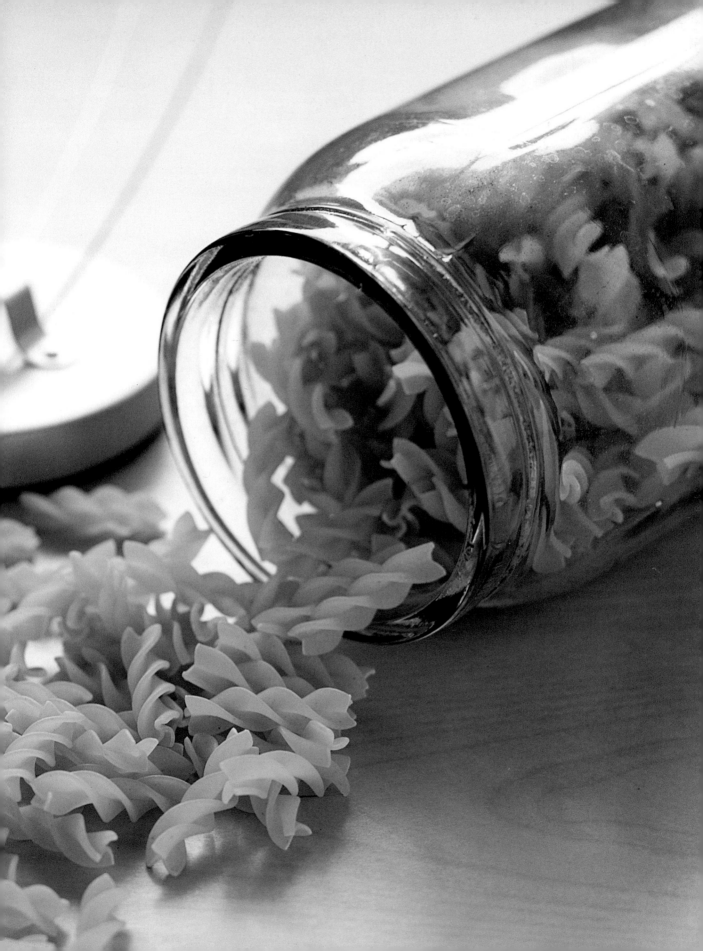

tofu
and vegetable noodle stir-fry

This tofu and vegetable stir-fry is packed full of colour, taste and texture, and it's filling enough to be a main course.

SERVES 4 Ⓥ ✳

Syns per serving
Original: 14½
Green: ½

Preparation time 10 minutes
Cooking time about 12 minutes

300g/11oz dried medium egg noodles

Fry Light

1 tsp sesame oil

2 garlic cloves, peeled and finely chopped

1 tsp peeled and finely grated ginger

1 red chilli, deseeded and finely chopped

6 spring onions, trimmed and cut into 1.5cm/¾in lengths

110g/4oz mangetout, halved lengthways

1 carrot, peeled and cut into thin matchsticks

400g/14oz firm tofu, cut into 1.5cm/¾in cubes

2 tbsp soy sauce

salt and freshly ground black pepper

a small handful of coriander leaves, chopped

1. Cook the noodles according to the packet instructions, drain and set aside.

2. Spray a large, non-stick wok or frying pan with Fry Light. Place over a medium heat and add the sesame oil, garlic, ginger, chilli, spring onions, mangetout and carrot. Stir-fry for 6–8 minutes or until the vegetables are just tender.

3. Add the tofu, soy sauce and the reserved noodles and toss to mix well. Stir-fry for 2–3 minutes and remove from the heat. Season well and stir in the coriander leaves just before serving.

mixed vegetable pad thai

Crunchy vegetables, bean sprouts and rice noodles flavoured with garlic, ginger, chilli and soy sauce make this a light and spicy lunch that's Free on the Green plan.

SERVES 4 ❋

Syns per serving
Original: 11½
Green: Free

Preparation time 10 minutes
Cooking time 12–15 minutes

Fry Light

2 garlic cloves, peeled and crushed

1 tsp peeled and finely grated ginger

1 red chilli, deseeded and finely chopped

8 spring onions, trimmed and cut into 1.5cm/¾in lengths

60ml/2fl oz chicken stock made with Bovril (or vegetable stock made with Vecon)

2 tbsp dark soy sauce

¼ tsp artificial sweetener (optional)

2 carrots, peeled and finely julienned

200g/7oz pak choi, roughly chopped

250g/9oz bean sprouts

250g/9oz dried medium rice noodles

1 egg, lightly beaten

To serve
sliced spring onion
chopped coriander leaves
lime wedges

1. Spray a large, non-stick wok or frying pan with Fry Light. Add the garlic, ginger, chilli, spring onions, stock, soy sauce and sweetener. Heat gently for 4–5 minutes.

2. Turn the heat to high and add the carrots, pak choi and bean sprouts. Stir-fry the vegetables for 4–5 minutes until they are just tender.

3. Prepare the noodles according to packet instructions, drain and add to the vegetable mixture in the frying pan over a high heat. Drizzle over the beaten egg and toss to mix well and cook for 1–2 minutes until the egg is just cooked through. Remove from the heat and sprinkle over the spring onions, coriander and a squeeze of lime juice before serving.

quick pasta 'cake'

Here's a quick pasta 'cake', filled with vegetables, herbs and spices that makes an ideal light lunch served with salad. It would be a fine addition to any picnic too!

SERVES 4 Ⓥ ❄

Syns per serving

With Parmesan

Original: 8

Green: 1

Without Parmesan

Original: 7

Green: Free

Preparation time 10 minutes

Cooking time about 20 minutes

Fry Light

6 spring onions, trimmed and finely sliced

2 garlic cloves, peeled and crushed

2 tomatoes, deseeded and finely chopped

1 red pepper, deseeded and finely diced

200g/7oz fresh or frozen peas

25g/1oz fresh basil leaves, chopped

400g/14oz cooked short-shape pasta, such as penne, fusilli, farfalle

6 eggs

4 tbsp chopped flat-leaf parsley

2 tbsp finely grated Parmesan cheese (optional)

salt and freshly ground black pepper

To serve

green salad

1. Spray a non-stick lidded frying pan with Fry Light and add the spring onions and garlic. Stir-fry over a medium heat for 1 minute and then add the tomatoes, red pepper and peas. Stir-fry for 4–5 minutes and then add the basil leaves and the cooked pasta.

2. Beat the eggs in a large bowl, stir in the chopped herbs and Parmesan cheese, if using. Season well and pour over the pasta mixture. Cover the pan and cook gently for 10 minutes or until the base is set.

3. Preheat the grill to medium-hot. Place the pan under the grill and cook for 4–5 minutes or until the top is set and golden. Remove and allow to sit for 5 minutes before carefully turning out onto a chopping board. Serve warm or cold, cut into wedges and with a crisp green salad.

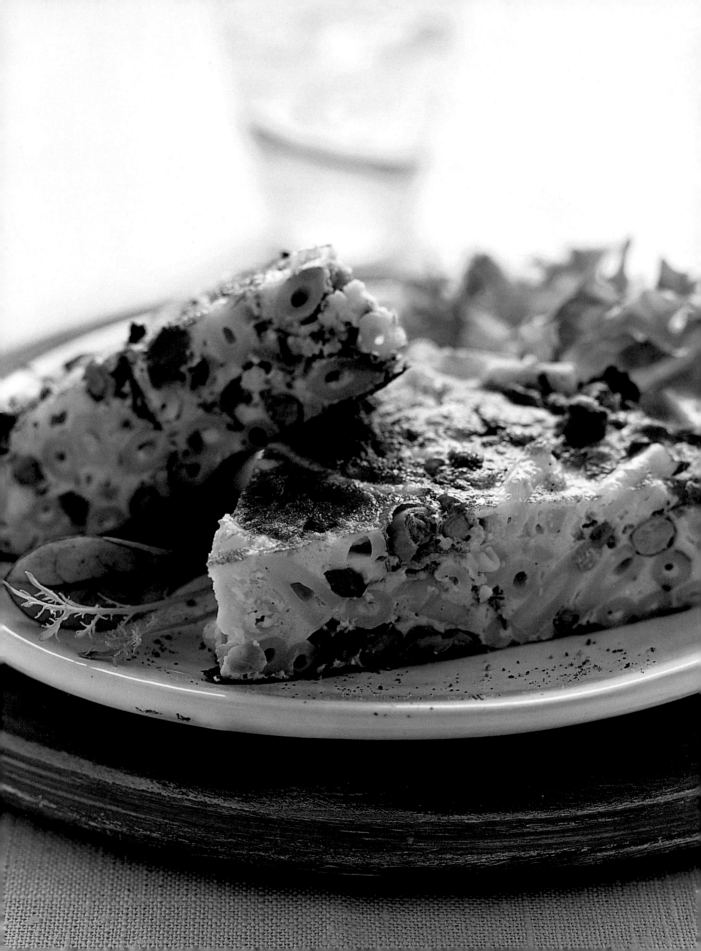

pasta napoletana

A quick and easy dish, here is fettucini tossed in a sauce of red onion, tomatoes, olives and herbs and served on a simple wild rocket salad.

SERVES 4 Ⓥ ❋
Syns per serving
Original: 15½
Green: ½

Preparation time 10 minutes
Cooking time about 15 minutes

350g/12oz dried fettucini
Fry Light
2 red onions, peeled, halved and thinly sliced
2 garlic cloves, peeled and sliced
400g can chopped tomatoes
1 tsp dried oregano
1–2 tsp artificial sweetener (optional)
salt and freshly ground black pepper
12 pitted black olives
4 tbsp roughly chopped basil leaves

To serve
basil leaves
wild rocket leaves

1. Cook the pasta in a large saucepan of lightly salted boiling water for 10–12 minutes or until just tender. Drain and keep warm.

2. While the pasta is cooking, spray a large, non-stick frying pan with Fry Light and place over a medium heat. Add the red onions and garlic and stir-fry for 2–3 minutes and then add the tomatoes, dried oregano and sweetener and bring to the boil. Reduce the heat, cover and gently simmer for 10 minutes. Season well and remove from the heat.

3. Transfer the mixture to a large, shallow serving platter. Stir in the olives and basil. Add the drained fettucini to the tomato mixture and toss to mix well. Serve immediately, garnished with basil leaves. Accompany with a wild rocket salad.

tomato, mushroom and pasta bake

This simple pasta bake is made with mushrooms, tomatoes and herbs, topped with cheese and grilled until cooked. Perfection on a plate!

SERVES 4 ❋

Syns per serving

With Cheddar

Original: 9½

Green: 4

Without Cheddar

Original: 5½

Green: Free

Preparation time 10 minutes

Cooking time about 20 minutes

Fry Light

1 onion, peeled and finely chopped

2 garlic cloves, peeled and finely chopped

400g/14oz mushrooms, finely chopped

400g can chopped tomatoes

90ml/3fl oz chicken stock made with Bovril

2 tsp dried oregano

6 tbsp chopped flat-leaf parsley

400g/14oz cooked short-shape pasta, such as penne, fusilli, farfalle

salt and freshly ground black pepper

110g/4oz reduced fat Cheddar cheese, grated (optional)

To serve

mixed salad

1. Preheat the oven to 200°C/Gas 6. Spray a large, non-stick frying pan with Fry Light and place over a high heat. Add the onion, garlic and mushrooms and stir-fry for 4–5 minutes.

2. Stir in the tomatoes, stock and dried oregano and bring to the boil. Remove from the heat and stir in the parsley and pasta and season well. Transfer to a shallow ovenproof dish, top with the cheese, if using, and bake in the oven for 8–10 minutes until hot and bubbling. Serve immediately with mixed salad leaves.

broccoli
and garlic pennette

Not for the faint-hearted, this quick to prepare, fiery pasta dish is perfect for a replenishing supper.

SERVES 4 Ⓥ ❄

Syns per serving

With Parmesan

Original: 12

Green: 1

Without Parmesan

Original: 11½

Green: Free

Preparation time 10 minutes

Cooking time about 10 minutes

400g/14oz broccoli, cut into florets

250g/9oz dried pennette or any other short-shape pasta, such as penne, fusilli, farfalle

Fry Light

4 garlic cloves, peeled and thinly sliced

1 tsp dried red chilli flakes

salt and freshly ground black pepper

To serve

2 tbsp grated Parmesan cheese (optional)

1. Blanch the broccoli in a large pan of lightly salted boiling water for 3–4 minutes. Drain and keep warm.

2. Cook the pasta in a large pan of lightly salted boiling water according to the packet instructions. Drain and keep warm.

3. While the pasta is cooking, spray a large, non-stick frying pan with Fry Light and place over a medium heat. Add the garlic, dried chilli flakes and broccoli and 90ml/3fl oz water. Stir and cook over a high heat for 3–4 minutes or until the broccoli is just tender, but still retains a slight bite.

4. Add the drained pennette to the mixture and stir over a high heat for 1–2 minutes and toss to mix well. Season and serve immediately sprinkled with grated Parmesan cheese, if using.

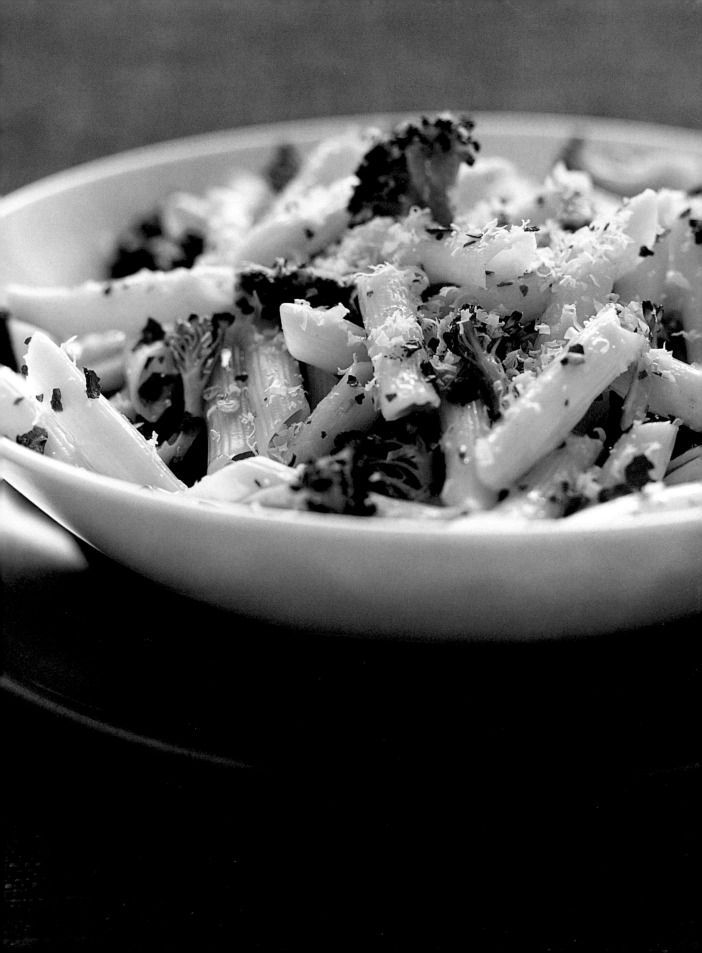

leek
and chive carbonara

**A tasty Green day version of pasta carbonara using leeks instead of ham –
and ready in only 20 minutes.**

SERVES 4 Ⓥ

Syns per serving
Original: 14½
Green: 1

Preparation time 10 minutes
Cooking time about 10 minutes

2 tbsp grated Parmesan
cheese

4 tbsp Quark soft cheese

110g/4oz very low fat natural
fromage frais

1 egg

4 tbsp chopped chives

salt and freshly ground black
pepper

300g/11oz dried spaghetti or
any other pasta of your choice

Fry Light

2 garlic cloves, peeled and
finely chopped

4 leeks, white parts only, finely
sliced

1. In a small bowl, mix the Parmesan and Quark cheeses with the fromage frais, egg, chives and a little salt and set aside.

2. Cook the pasta according to the packet instructions. Drain and set aside.

3. While the pasta is cooking, heat some Fry Light in a large, non-stick frying pan and cook the garlic for 1–2 minutes until lightly browned.

4. At the same time, steam the leeks for 4–5 minutes until softened. Stir into the frying pan with the garlic and cook for 2–3 minutes over a high heat. Add the cheese mixture, remove from the heat, and stir for 1–2 minutes.

5. Pour over the reserved pasta and quickly mix through, season well and serve immediately.

mixed mushroom and pasta gratin

In this simple version of an Italian classic, mushrooms are cooked with tomatoes, spring onions and garlic, tossed with cooked pasta and finished off with a creamy mustard mozzarella topping.

SERVES 4 Ⓥ ❋

Syns per serving

With mozzarella

Original: 8

Green: 2½

Without mozzarella

Original: 5½

Green: Free

Preparation time 6–8 minutes

Cooking time about 22 minutes

Fry Light

6 spring onions, trimmed and thinly sliced

2 garlic cloves, peeled and chopped

450g/1lb mixed mushrooms, halved or quartered

6 plum tomatoes, roughly chopped

salt and freshly ground black pepper

400g/14oz cooked short-shape pasta, such as penne, fusilli, farfalle

For the topping

500g/1lb 2oz very low fat natural yogurt

1 tsp Dijon mustard

110g/4oz reduced fat mozzarella cheese, coarsely grated (optional)

2 eggs, lightly beaten

1. Spray a large, non-stick frying pan with Fry Light and place over a high heat. Add the spring onions, garlic and mushrooms and stir and cook for 2–3 minutes. Add 90ml/3fl oz water to the pan and cook for 4–5 minutes until the water has been absorbed.

2. Stir in the tomatoes, season well and add the cooked pasta. Toss to mix well. Transfer this mixture to a shallow, ovenproof dish.

3. Preheat the oven to 180°C/Gas 4. Make the topping by mixing all the ingredients in a bowl. Season well and pour over the pasta mixture. Place in the oven and cook for 10–15 minutes or until lightly golden and bubbly. Remove, let stand for 5 minutes before serving. Accompany with mixed salad leaves or steamed green vegetables.

lemon, courgette
and minted pea fusilli

Lemon and mint add a zing to this creamy, filling dish of fusilli pasta, courgettes and peas.

SERVES 4 Ⓥ ❄

Syns per serving
Original: 17
Green: Free

Preparation time 10–12 minutes
Cooking time 8–10 minutes

350g/12oz dried fusilli or any other short-shape pasta, such as penne, farfalle

Fry Light

2 garlic cloves, peeled and crushed

4 spring onions, trimmed and finely chopped

2 courgettes, roughly grated

200g/7oz fresh or frozen peas

250g/9oz very low fat natural fromage frais

finely grated zest of 1 lemon

a small handful of mint leaves, finely chopped

salt and freshly ground black pepper

1. Cook the pasta in a large saucepan of lightly salted boiling water for 10–12 minutes or until just tender. Drain and keep warm.

2. Spray a large, non-stick frying pan with Fry Light and place over a medium heat. Add the garlic and spring onions and stir-fry for 2–3 minutes. Turn the heat to high and add the courgettes and peas. Stir and cook for a further 4–5 minutes or until the courgette has softened.

3. Reduce the heat to low and stir in the fromage frais, lemon zest and mint. Add the drained pasta to the mixture, season and toss to mix well. Serve immediately, ladled into warmed bowls.

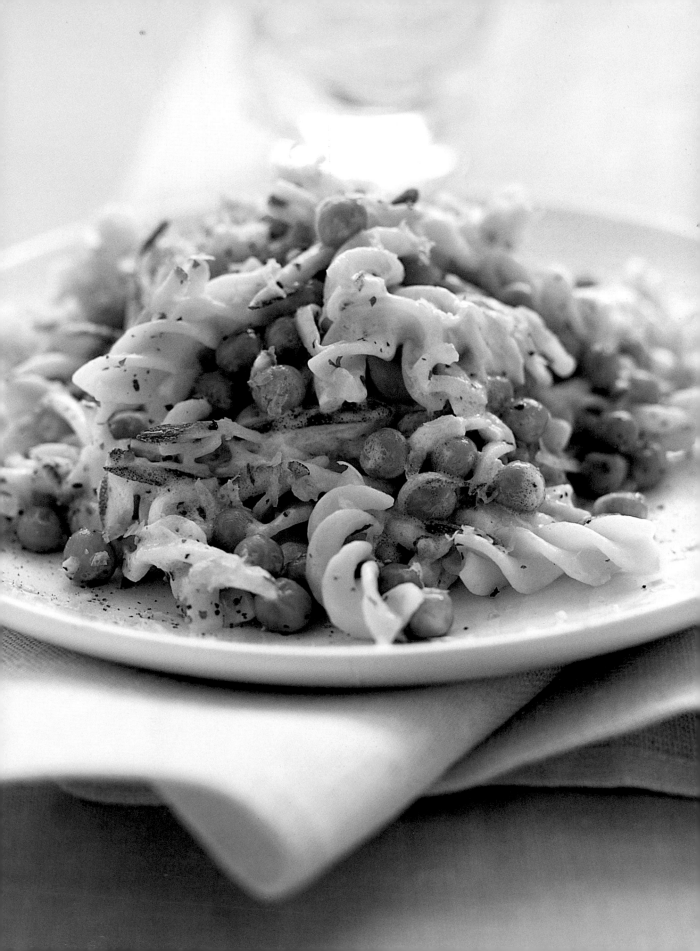

individual
vegetable lasagnes

If you're in the mood to cook up a treat, follow these five easy steps to create individual vegetable lasagnes that would grace any dinner table.

SERVES 4 Ⓥ ❋

Syns per serving
With Parmesan
Original: 11
Green: 6

Without Parmesan
Original: 5
Green: Free

Preparation time 10 minutes
Cooking time about 20–25 minutes

Fry Light

3 garlic cloves, peeled and crushed

350g/12oz Quorn mince

1 small aubergine, finely diced

1 courgette, finely diced

1 red pepper, deseeded and finely diced

1 red onion, peeled and finely diced

salt and freshly ground black pepper

200g/7oz very low fat natural yogurt

250g/9oz Quark soft cheese

a large pinch of ground nutmeg

2 x 400g cans chopped tomatoes

2 tsp dried mixed herbs

8 pre-cooked lasagne sheets

110g/4oz Parmesan cheese, grated (optional)

To serve

green salad

1. Preheat the oven to 220°C/Gas 7. Spray a large, non-stick frying pan with Fry Light and place over a high heat. Add the garlic, Quorn and vegetables. Season well and then stir-fry for 2–3 minutes.

2. In a bowl, whisk the yogurt with the Quark, nutmeg and chopped tomatoes until well combined. Season and stir in the dried herbs.

3. Spray four individual ovenproof dishes with Fry Light. Spoon half the vegetable and Quorn mixture to cover the bases and cover with half the lasagne sheets. Top with half the creamy tomato/Quark sauce.

4. Layer the rest of the vegetables on top and cover with the remaining pasta sheets and the sauce. Sprinkle over the grated Parmesan cheese, if using, and bake for 15–20 minutes or until lightly browned.

5. Remove from the oven and allow to cool for 5–10 minutes before serving accompanied by a crisp green salad.

basil and chilli linguine

In a hurry? Need something tasty, hot and filling? This quick-and-easy basil and chilli linguine fits the bill on all counts.

SERVES 4 Ⓥ ❋

Syns per serving

With Parmesan

Original: 23½

Green: 1

Without Parmesan

Original: 22½

Green: Free

Preparation time 6–8 minutes

Cooking time about 15 minutes

500g/1lb 2oz dried quick-cook linguine or spaghetti

Fry Light

1 onion, peeled and finely chopped

2 garlic cloves, peeled and finely sliced

400g can chopped tomatoes

1 tsp dried chilli flakes

¼ tsp artificial sweetener

a large handful of basil leaves, chopped

salt and freshly ground black pepper

To serve

2 tbsp grated Parmesan cheese (optional)

1. Cook the pasta in a large saucepan of lightly salted boiling water until just tender. Drain and keep warm.

2. While the pasta is cooking, spray a large, non-stick frying pan with Fry Light and add the onion and garlic. Stir and cook for 3–4 minutes and then add the tomatoes, chilli and sweetener. Turn the heat to high and bring to the boil. Reduce the heat to medium, cover and cook gently for 8–10 minutes, stirring occasionally to prevent sticking.

3. Remove from the heat and stir in the chopped basil, season well, and serve with the drained pasta, sprinkling some Parmesan on, if using, just before serving.

mexican
vegetable rice

This substantial colourful rice dish makes a fabulous Green day main course. Plus, it's fast – and it's Free.

SERVES 4 Ⓥ ❄

Syns per serving
Original: 21½
Green: Free

Preparation time 5 minutes
Cooking time about 15 minutes

Fry Light

1 onion, peeled and finely chopped

1 garlic clove, peeled and finely chopped

1 tsp ground cumin

½ red pepper, deseeded and finely diced

200g/7oz cherry tomatoes, halved

400g can red kidney beans, drained and rinsed

400g can sweetcorn kernels, drained and rinsed

200g/7oz fresh or frozen peas

500g/1lb 2oz cooked white or brown basmati rice

salt and freshly ground black pepper

1. Spray a large, non-stick frying pan with Fry Light and place over a medium heat. Add the onion, garlic, cumin and red pepper and stir-fry for 4–5 minutes.

2. Stir in the tomatoes, red kidney beans, sweetcorn and peas, turn the heat to high and stir-fry for 3–4 minutes.

3. Stir in the rice and toss to mix well. Stir and cook for 3–4 minutes until piping hot. Remove from the heat and season well. Serve immediately.

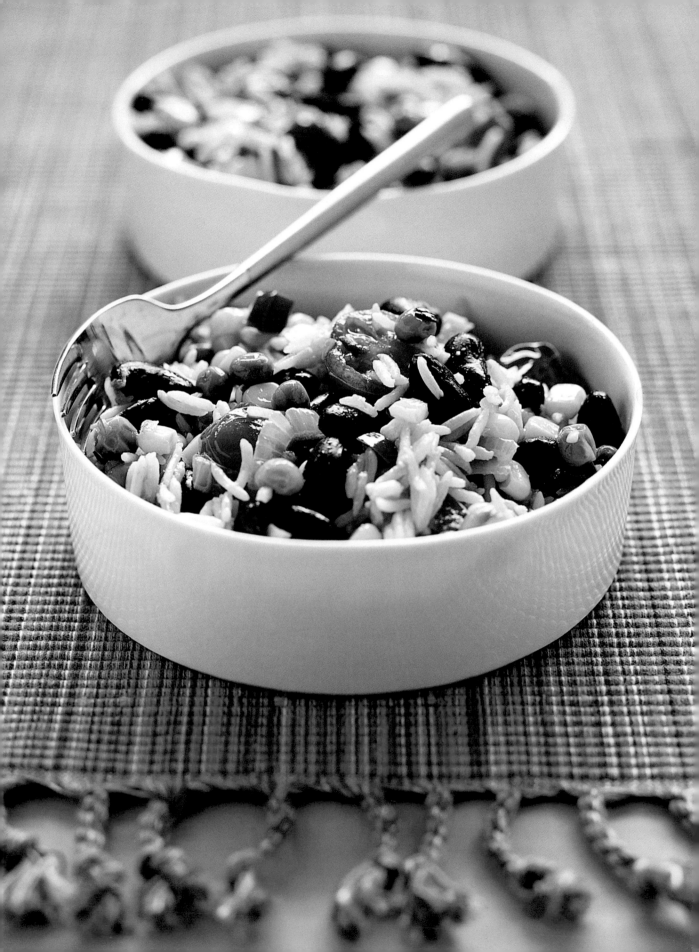

indonesian-style quick fried rice

The vegetables for this recipe can be varied endlessly according to what you have in, so this dish is always fresh and different.

SERVES 4 Ⓥ ❄

Syns per serving
Original: 7
Green: Free

Preparation time 10 minutes
Cooking time 10–12 minutes

1 courgette, cut into thick batons

1 carrot, peeled and cut into thin matchsticks

200g/7oz fine beans, trimmed and cut in half

Fry Light

6 spring onions, trimmed and finely sliced on the diagonal

3 garlic cloves, peeled and thinly sliced

1 tsp ground coriander

1 tsp medium curry powder

1 red pepper, deseeded and cut into thin strips

400g/14oz cooked and cooled white rice

2 tbsp light soy sauce

salt and freshly ground black pepper

2 eggs

1 tbsp finely chopped coriander leaves

1 tbsp water

To garnish
chopped coriander and mint leaves

1. Blanch the courgette, carrot and beans in a large pan of boiling water for 2 minutes, drain and set aside.

2. Spray a large frying pan with Fry Light and add the spring onions, garlic, ground coriander and curry powder. Stir-fry for 2–3 minutes and then add the red pepper. Stir-fry for another minute and then add the rice, courgette, carrots and beans. Stir-fry for 3–4 minutes and then stir in the soy sauce. Toss to mix well, season, remove from the heat, cover and keep hot.

3. Spray a non-stick frying pan with Fry Light and place over a low heat. Beat the eggs in a bowl with the coriander leaves and water. Pour the egg mixture into the pan and rotate to cover the base of the pan evenly. Cook gently for 1–2 minutes or until the base is set and then carefully turn over and cook for another minute. Turn out onto a work surface and cut the omelette into thin strips.

4. To serve, divide the rice mixture between four warmed serving plates or bowls and top with the herbed omelette strips. Serve immediately, garnished with coriander and mint leaves.

asparagus and leek risotto

Here is a wonderfully creamy risotto made with fresh asparagus and leeks and topped with a tangy soft cheese.

SERVES 4 Ⓥ ❄

Syns per serving
Original: 11½
Green: Free

Preparation time 5 minutes
Cooking time about 25 minutes

Fry Light

8–10 spring onions, trimmed and finely chopped

2 garlic cloves, peeled and finely chopped

6 baby leeks, white parts only, finely sliced

1 carrot, peeled and finely diced

250g/9oz dried Arborio or risotto rice

900ml/1½ pints boiling water or vegetable stock made with Vecon

400g/14oz asparagus tips, trimmed

salt and freshly ground black pepper

6 tbsp chopped flat-leaf parsley

1 tbsp chopped tarragon

110g/4oz Quark soft cheese (optional)

1. Spray a large, non-stick frying pan with Fry Light and place over a medium heat. Add the spring onions, garlic, leeks, carrot and rice and stir-fry for 1–2 minutes.

2. Add a large ladleful of the boiling water or stock and stir and cook until the liquid is absorbed. Repeat, adding a ladleful at a time, until half the stock is used up.

3. Stir in the asparagus and continue to cook the risotto in this manner until all the stock is used up and the rice is creamy and al dente (tender but still retaining a bite). This should take about 18–20 minutes.

4. Remove from the heat, season well and stir in the chopped herbs. Ladle into individual warmed pasta bowls, spoon over the Quark, if using, and serve immediately.

creamy pumpkin risotto

This brightly coloured dish of golden-orange pumpkin, red onion and tomato makes a substantial supper for four.

SERVES 4 Ⓥ ❄

Syns per serving
Original: 9
Green: Free

Preparation time 10 minutes
Cooking time about 15 minutes

500g/1lb 2oz pumpkin, cut into 1cm/½in dice

1 red onion, finely chopped

2 garlic cloves, finely chopped

300ml/½ pint vegetable stock made with Vecon

500g/1lb 2oz cooked brown or white basmati rice

6 plum tomatoes, finely chopped

2 tsp dried mixed herbs

salt and freshly ground black pepper

110g/4oz very low fat natural fromage frais

4 tbsp finely chopped flat-leaf parsley

1. Place the pumpkin, red onion and garlic in a large, non-stick frying pan with the stock and bring to the boil. Cover and simmer gently for 8–10 minutes or until the pumpkin is just tender.

2. Stir in the rice, tomatoes and dried herbs. Season well and stir and cook for 3–4 minutes or until the mixture is piping hot.

3. Remove from the heat, stir in the fromage frais and parsley and serve immediately, ladled into warmed bowls or plates.

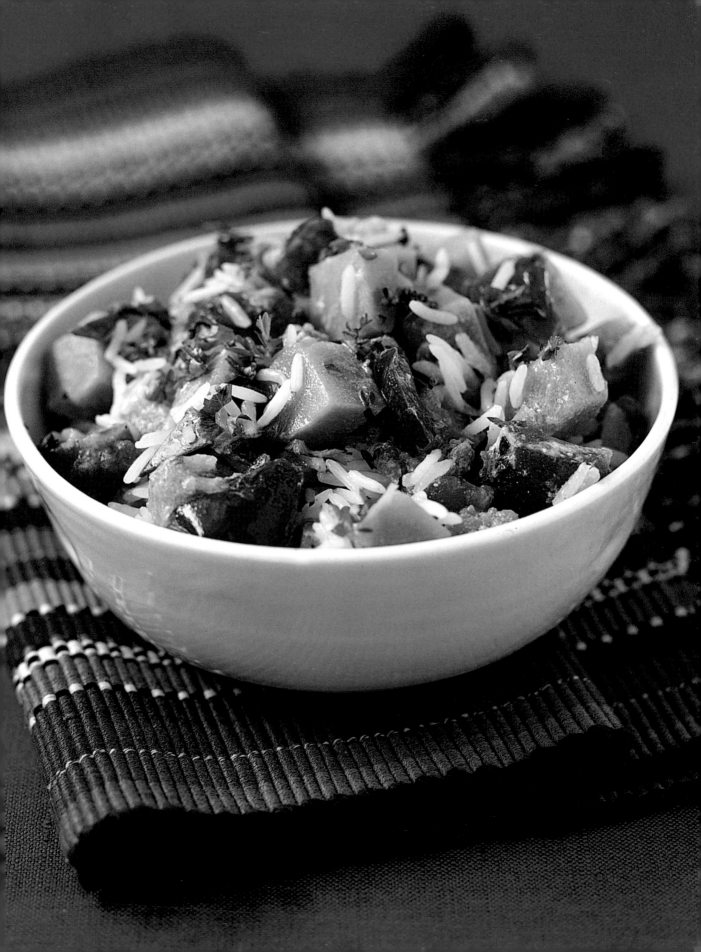

quinoa and vegetable 'pilaff'

Quinoa (pronounced keen-wa) is a super-grain that was grown by the Aztecs in South America. It is now widely sold in supermarkets and organic grocery and health food stores and can be used in a variety of dishes.

SERVES 4 Ⓥ ❄

Syns per serving
Original: 12½
Green: Free

Preparation time 10 minutes
Cooking time about 18 minutes

300g/11oz quinoa

Fry Light

2 garlic cloves, peeled and finely chopped

6 spring onions, trimmed and thinly sliced

2 red peppers, deseeded and finely diced

1 yellow pepper, deseeded and finely diced

1 courgette, finely diced

200ml/7fl oz boiling water or vegetable stock made with Vecon

4 tbsp finely chopped basil leaves

4 tbsp finely chopped flat-leaf parsley

salt and freshly ground black pepper

1. In a bowl, prepare the quinoa according to the packet instructions and set aside.

2. Spray a large, non-stick frying pan with Fry Light and place over a medium heat. Add the garlic, spring onions, red and yellow peppers and courgette and stir-fry for 6–8 minutes.

3. Add the water or stock and continue to cook for 5–6 minutes or until most of the water or stock is absorbed. Add the reserved quinoa and stir and cook for 2–3 minutes.

4. Remove from the heat and add the chopped herbs. Season well and serve immediately.

lemon-roasted
vegetable couscous

Couscous and roasted vegetables are perfect dinner partners. The addition of lemon gives the dish an extra kick.

SERVES 4 ❀
Syns per serving
Original: 14
Green: Free

Preparation time 10 minutes
Cooking time about 20 minutes

Fry Light

2 red peppers, deseeded and cut into 2.5cm/1in pieces

1 aubergine, cut into 2.5cm/1in cubes

2 red onions, peeled and cut into thick wedges

2 courgettes, cut into 2.5cm/1in cubes

200g/7oz cherry tomatoes

salt and freshly ground black pepper

300g/11oz dried couscous

1 tbsp finely chopped preserved lemon

1 tsp ground ginger

1 tsp ground cinnamon

1 tsp ground cumin

juice of 1 lemon

60ml/2fl oz chicken stock made with Bovril (or vegetable stock made with Vecon)

a handful of coriander leaves, chopped

a handful of mint leaves, chopped

1. Preheat the oven to 220°C/Gas 7. Spray a large, non-stick roasting tin with Fry Light and spread the vegetables onto it in a single layer. (If there are too many, then use a second roasting tin.) Spray the vegetables with Fry Light and season well. Roast in the oven for 20 minutes or until cooked and lightly charred at the edges. Remove from the heat.

2. Meanwhile, make up the couscous according to the packet instructions. In a bowl, mix together the preserved lemon, ginger, cinnamon, cumin, lemon juice and stock. Stir this into the couscous with a fork and then add the roasted vegetables and the roasting juices from the tin. Toss gently with a fork to mix, add the chopped herbs and serve immediately. This dish is equally good when served at room temperature and makes a great lunchbox filler.

mixed bean
and barley stew

This filling, satisfying mixed bean and barley stew is the perfect way to warm up on a cold winter's day.

SERVES 4 ⓥ ❋

Syns per serving
Original: 17
Green: Free

Preparation time 5 minutes
Cooking time about 20 minutes

Fry Light

2 garlic cloves, peeled and finely chopped

1 tbsp chopped rosemary leaves

400g can chopped tomatoes

200ml/7fl oz boiling water or vegetable stock made with Vecon

400g can borlotti beans, drained and rinsed

400g can cannellini beans, drained and rinsed

400g can chickpeas, drained and rinsed

200g/7oz cooked barley

salt and freshly ground black pepper

1. Spray a large, non-stick frying pan with Fry Light. Place over a medium heat and add the garlic and rosemary. Stir-fry for 1 minute and then add the tomatoes, water or stock, beans, chickpeas and barley. Bring to the boil, cover tightly and reduce the heat to medium-low. Cook gently for 20 minutes.

2. Remove the bean stew from the heat, season well and serve ladled into warm bowls.

tip
You can cook the barley the day before. Just boil in a large pan of boiling water for 20 minutes.

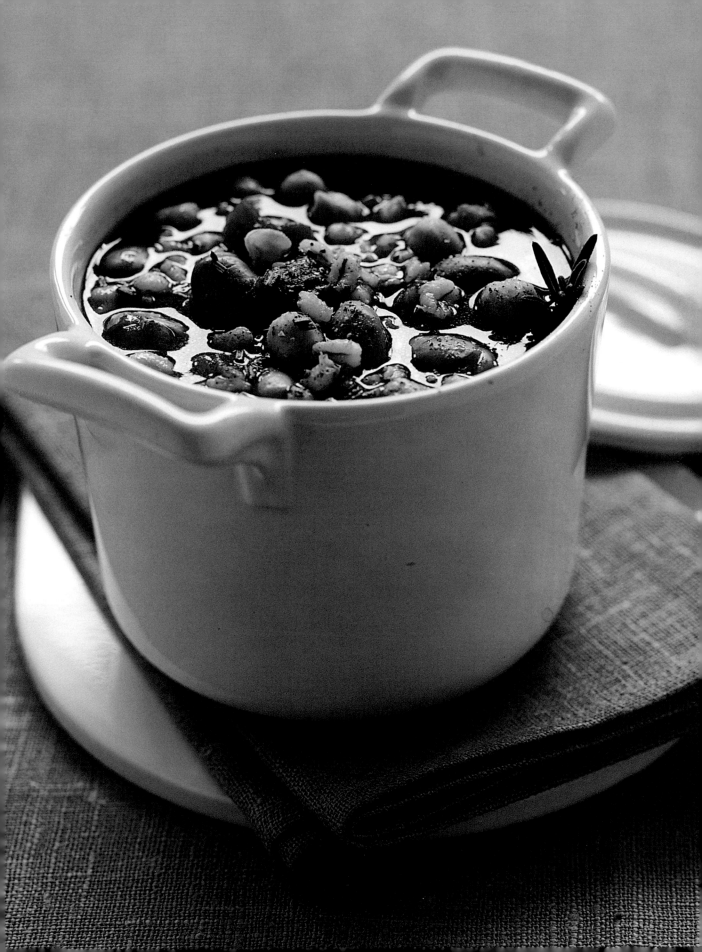

happiness
by the forkful!

Fork-lift truck drivers Neil and Kathy Feeley live in Barnsley, south Yorkshire, with their teenage daughter Rachel. The couple were voted Mr and Mrs Slimming World 2004.

Life has changed out of all recognition for fork-lift truck drivers Neil and Kathy Feeley since they lost a mammoth 13st 4lb between them.

At one time Neil, whose weight peaked at 20st, and Kathy, who topped 16½st, struggled to squeeze behind the controls of their fork-lifts and despite a wonderfully happy marriage, found their social life restricted and their daughter the target of school bullies.

Since losing the weight, the couple say they have fallen in love all over again. Their plans for Kathy's 40th birthday celebrations featured a renewal of their wedding vows on a tropical beach with Kathy wearing a slinky size 12 dress.

It's a far cry from the size 24 'meringue-like' dress Kathy had to don for their wedding in 1987. The couple soon settled into a blissful family life in which food played a major role. A diet full of high-fat home-cooked meals, takeaways and pub dinners eventually took its toll on the couple's confidence and health.

The turning point came when doctors told Kathy a minor operation she needed would be too risky because of her size. Though Kathy argued for six months against Neil's suggestion they join their local Slimming World group, she finally agreed – and was delighted to find her fears of public humiliation were unfounded.

Both Neil and Kathy were thrilled to discover that no foods were 'off limits'. It made all the difference to lose weight without sacrificing family meals such as spaghetti bolognese, egg and chips and shepherd's pie – and Food Optimising fitted so easily into their lifestyle. Neil was happy to forego his usual full English breakfast in the canteen, opting to take his own bread and enjoy a large grilled bacon sandwich instead.

And he's not the only Feeley to enjoy their new food freedom. Neil confided: 'Our daughter Rachel enjoys more and more of the foods we're eating. She particularly likes Syn-free chips and she loves Slimming World quiche. If I make a shepherd's pie with Quorn, which she wouldn't normally dream of eating, she has no idea it isn't meat and she really enjoys it.

'The great thing is that we're not just influencing Rachel's eating choices, we've influenced lots of friends, including one who lost 6st with Slimming World. Colleagues often say: "How can you be on a diet and be eating that?" but I just tell them I'm not on a diet. This way of eating is in our blood now.'

After struggling to squeeze behind the controls of their fork-lift trucks, Neil and Kathy have also discovered Body Magic and through it, a shared love of keep fit, even converting their garage into a home gym.

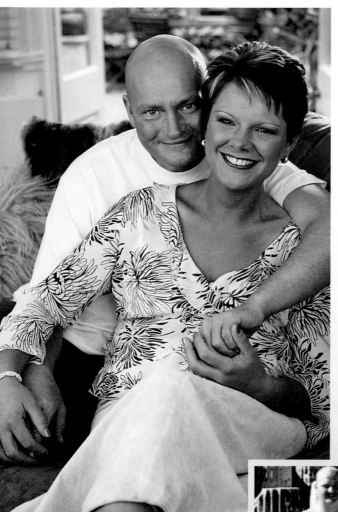

take **charge** of your thoughts

The one thing you have total control of is your thinking. Use it for your own benefit. Bombard your mind with thoughts, words, pictures and people that reaffirm the person you want to be and the things you want to achieve. Focus always on the things you want, not the things you fear or need to overcome. Your life today is the result of past choices. Your future depends on the choices you make today.

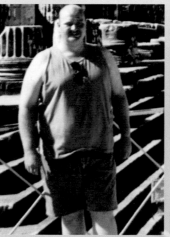

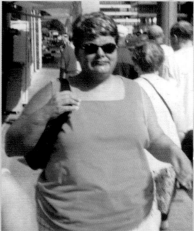

"We used to put some real rubbish in our mouths but since we started Food Optimising, we've never looked back and we can still enjoy the things we love, such as buffets and curries. Not only that, our daughter Rachel enjoys more and more of the foods we're eating."

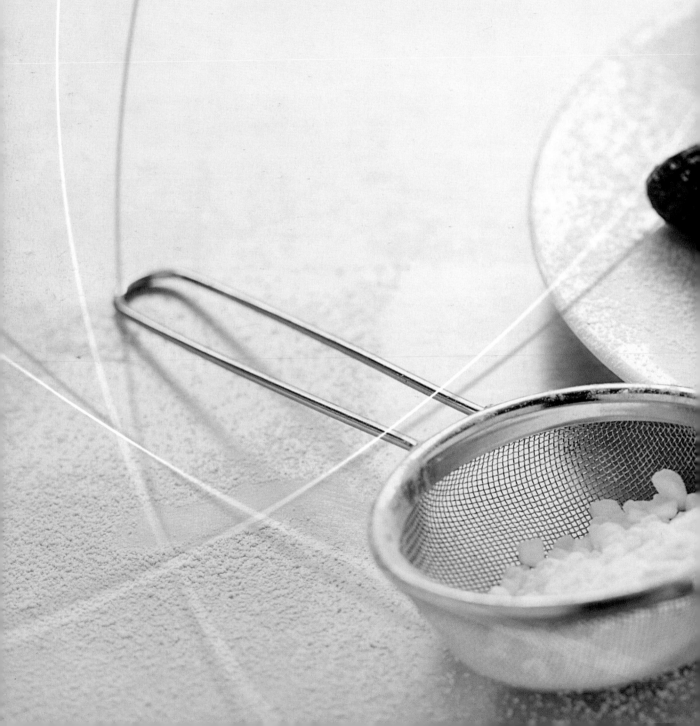

desserts

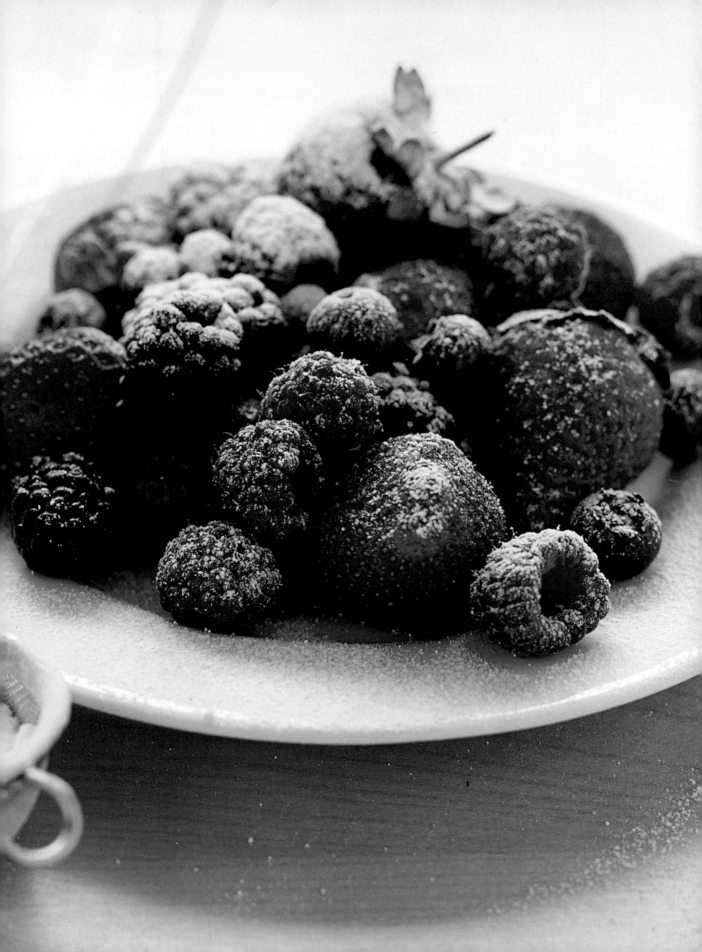

mango possets

Juicy orange mangoes snuggle beneath a light and frothy topping. Simplicity itself!

SERVES 4 ⓥ
Syns per serving
Original: 4½
Green: 4½

Preparation time 10 minutes
plus chilling

4 large mangoes
1 tbsp lemon juice
2 egg whites
2 tbsp artificial sweetener

1. Peel, stone and roughly chop the mango flesh, place in a blender with the lemon juice and process until smooth. Place a tablespoon or two of the purée in the bottom of four chilled dessert bowls, transfer the rest to a large bowl and set aside.

2. In a separate bowl, whisk the egg whites until softly peaked and then gradually whisk in the sweetener until the mixture is shiny and stiff.

3. Carefully fold the egg white mixture into the remaining mango and lemon purée until well combined and then spoon this into the dessert bowls. Chill in the fridge for 2–3 hours before serving.

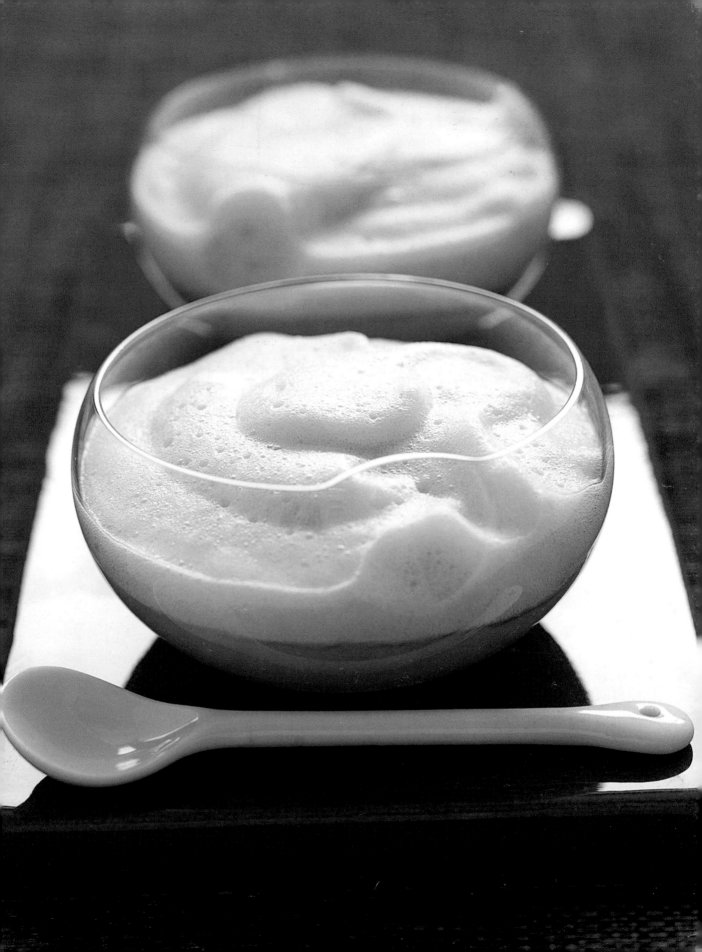

griddled pineapple
and nectarine skewers

Skewered fruits, grilled until lightly caramelised, make a dessert that is unusual yet easy – not to mention delicious!

SERVES 4 Ⓥ

Syns per serving
With sugar
Original: 6
Green: 6

Without sugar
Original: 5½
Green: 5½

Preparation time 10 minutes
Cooking time 4–5 minutes

1 small pineapple
(approximately 800g/1lb 12oz)
2 large nectarines
1 tbsp caster sugar (optional)

To decorate
chopped mint leaves

1. Peel, core and cut the pineapple into bite-sized pieces. Cut the nectarines into wedges. Thread the fruit alternately onto 8–12 pre-soaked bamboo skewers.

2. Preheat the grill to hot. Sprinkle the fruit with the sugar, if using, and place under the grill for 4–5 minutes, turning once. Alternatively, you can cook the skewers on a very hot, non-stick, ridged griddle pan.

3. Sprinkle the skewers with the mint leaves and serve them immediately.

lemon cheesecake filo tartlets

These lemon cheesecake filo tartlets make a light and fruity dessert. Fill the cases just before serving to prevent them softening.

MAKES 4 Ⓥ

Syns per serving
Original: 4½
Green: 4½

Preparation time 10 minutes
Cooking time 12–15 minutes

4 x 25g/1oz fresh filo pastry sheets
Fry Light

For cheesecake filling
150g/5oz Quark soft cheese
finely grated zest of 1 lemon
1 tbsp lemon juice
4 tbsp Müllerlight lemon cheesecake yogurt
1 tbsp artificial sweetener

To serve
lime zest
½ tsp icing sugar

1. Preheat the oven to 180°C/Gas 4. Cut the filo pastry into 12 squares (10 x 10cm/4 x 4in each). Lay them out on a clean work surface and spray with Fry Light. Lay one piece of pastry in the base of each of four individual tartlet cases. Repeat with the remaining pieces to form four tartlet cases, positioning each layer at a slightly different angle. Place in the oven and bake for 12–15 minutes or until golden brown and crisp. Remove and allow to cool.

2. Meanwhile, make the cheesecake filling by beating the Quark until smooth. Stir in the lemon zest and juice, Müllerlight yogurt and sweetener. Cover and chill until ready to serve.

3. To serve, spoon the cheese mixture into the filo cases. Decorate with lime zest and lightly dust with icing sugar before serving.

mixed berry jellies

Simple yet elegant, these individual mixed berry jellies will be a hit with children and adults alike. You can use any combination of fruit and flavoured jelly.

SERVES 4 ⓥ

Syns per serving
Original: 1
Green: 1

Preparation time 10 minutes
plus chilling

300g/11oz mixed summer berries

2 x 14g sachets sugar-free lemon-flavoured jelly

To serve
4 tbsp fat-free natural yogurt

1. Divide the mixed berries between four large dessert tumblers. Put in the fridge to chill.

2. Make the jelly according to the packet instructions and, when cool, pour over the prepared tumblers. Place in the fridge and chill for 5–6 hours or until just set.

3. Serve with the yogurt in a bowl alongside.

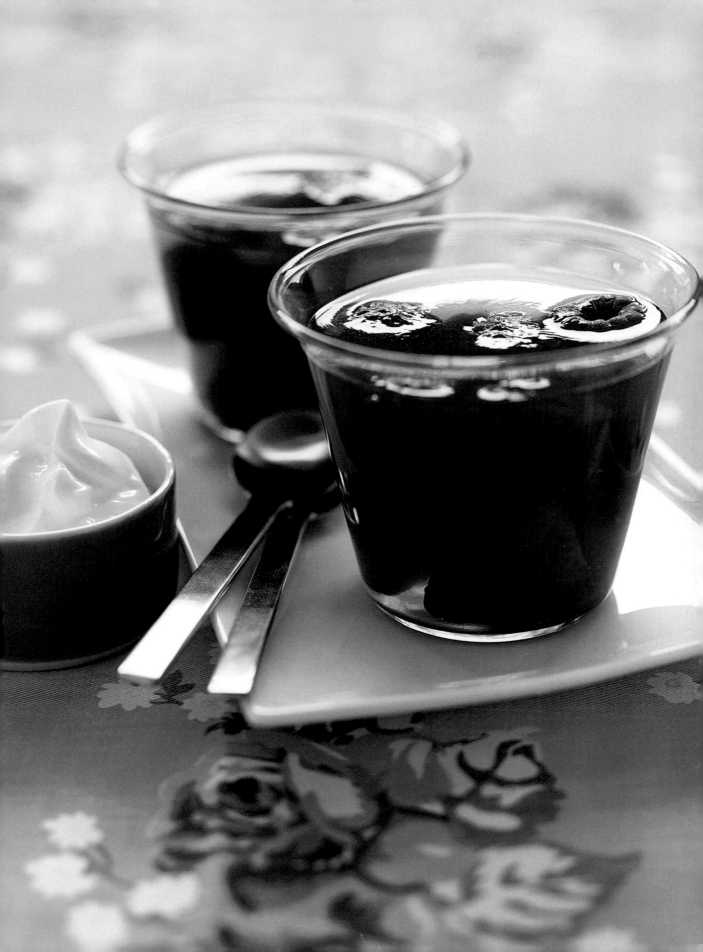

grape and blackcurrant pots

Good old jelly and custard given a grown-up twist.

SERVES 4 Ⓥ

Syns per serving

With custard

Original: 2

Green: 2

Without custard

Original: 1

Green: 1

Preparation time 10 minutes
plus chilling

2 x 14g sugar-free
blackcurrant jelly

300g/11oz mixed seedless
grapes

To serve

8 tbsp low fat custard
(optional) or Müllerlight vanilla
yogurt

1. Make the jelly according to the packet instructions. Set aside.

2. Divide the grapes between four individual jelly moulds or ramekins. Pour over the jelly and chill in the fridge until set.

3. When ready to serve, dip the moulds in hot water for a couple of seconds and turn out onto individual serving plates. Serve chilled with low fat custard, if using, or the Müllerlight yogurt.

peach and raspberry salad
with basil 'cream'

Fresh fruit with basil cream might sound a strange combination, but the flavours complement each other perfectly.

SERVES 4 Ⓥ

Syns per serving
Original: Free
Green: Free

Preparation time 10 minutes

4 peaches
300g/11oz raspberries
juice of 1 lemon
1 tsp artificial sweetener

For the 'cream'
300g/11oz very low fat natural fromage frais
2 tsp artificial sweetener
2 tbsp very finely chopped basil leaves

To decorate
basil leaves

1. Halve, stone and slice the peaches and place in a shallow dish with the raspberries.

2. Mix the lemon juice and sweetener and add to the fruit mixture. Toss to mix well.

3. To make the 'cream', mix together the fromage frais, sweetener and chopped basil and stir to mix well.

4. Serve the salad in bowls with a dollop of the cream and decorated with basil leaves.

berry puff tarts

**The reaction when you place these on the table will be a resounding 'Wow!'
They taste as good as they look too!**

MAKES 4 ⓥ

Syns per serving
Original: 6
Green: 6

Preparation time 10 minutes
Cooking time 12–15 minutes

110g/4oz bought puff pastry

For the filling
110g/4oz very low fat natural
fromage frais
50g/2oz Quark soft cheese
2 tbsp artificial sweetener
a few drops rose water

To serve
350g/12oz mixed berries
(preferably fresh)
½ tsp icing sugar

1. Preheat the oven to 220°C/Gas 7. Prepare a baking sheet by lining it with baking parchment. Divide the pastry into four equal portions and roll each one into a square approximately 8–10cm/4–5in. Place on the prepared baking sheet, well spaced apart.

2. With a sharp knife, score a border, about 5mm/¼in in along the edge of the pastry. Place in the oven and bake for 12–15 minutes until the pastry has risen slightly and is golden. Remove from the oven and cool on wire racks.

3. Meanwhile, make the filling. Beat together the fromage frais, Quark and sweetener. Flavour with the rose water. Push down the centres of the tarts to make space for the filling and carefully spoon onto the puff-pastry shells. Top with the berries and serve dusted with icing sugar.

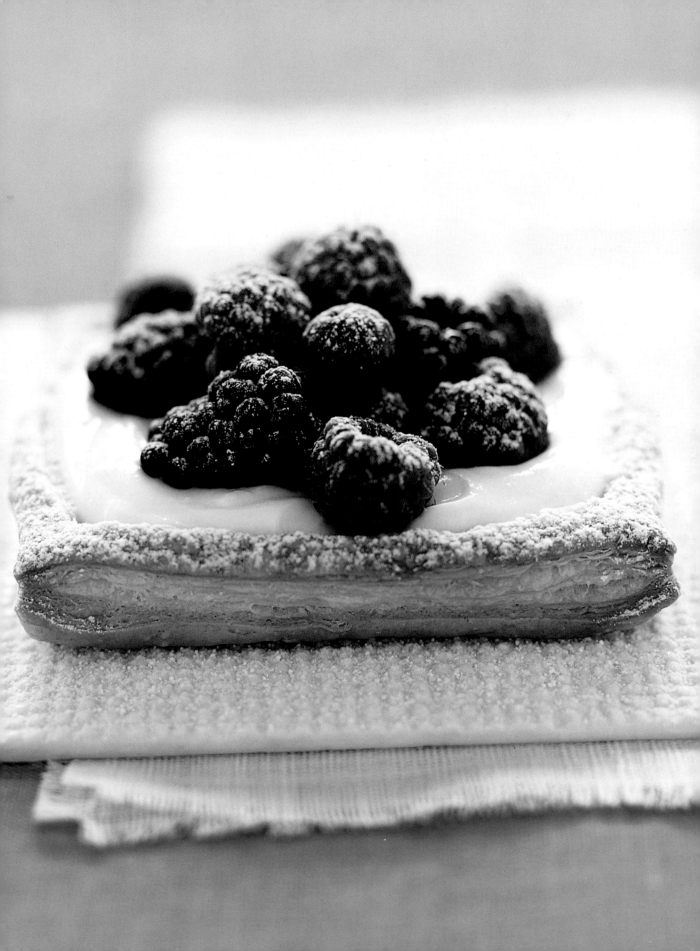

floating islands

The preparation of this dessert might seem a little fiddly, but the result is well worth the effort.

SERVES 4 ⓥ

Syns per serving
Original: 2½
Green: 2½

Preparation time 10 minutes
Cooking time about 5 minutes
per batch

For the mixed berry coulis
400g/14oz frozen mixed
berries, thawed
1 tbsp artificial sweetener

For the 'islands'
3 eggs, separated
3–4 tbsp granulated artificial
sweetener (or to taste)
90ml/3fl oz skimmed milk
200ml/7fl oz water
a few drops vanilla essence
1–2 tsp artificial sweetener

To decorate
½ tsp icing sugar
fresh berries (optional)
chopped mint leaves (optional)

1. To make the coulis, place the ingredients in a blender and process until smooth. Remove and set aside (you can use a fine metal sieve to strain the coulis if desired).

2. Whisk the egg whites in a clean, grease-free bowl with an electric whisk until firm. Gradually add the granulated sweetener and continue whisking until shiny and stiff.

3. Place the milk, water, vanilla and sweetener in a frying pan and bring to a gentle simmer. Using two dessertspoons, shape the meringue mixture into 12 egg shapes and gently lower, in batches, into the simmering liquid. Poach each batch for about 5 minutes until firm to the touch, turning once during cooking. (Be careful, as they are delicate and can disintegrate easily). Remove with a slotted spoon and set aside.

4. To serve, spoon the coulis onto the base of four soup plates and top each serving with three floating islands. Dust with icing sugar and decorate with berries and mint leaves, if desired.

amaretti stuffed nectarines

This is a brilliant way to serve nectarines when they're in season. Simply stuff the nectarine halves with the crushed biscuits mixed with soft cheese and almond liqueur.

SERVES 4 Ⓥ

Syns per serving
With Amaretto
Original: 1
Green: 1

Without Amaretto
Original: ½
Green: ½

Preparation time 10 minutes

6 nectarines
200g/7oz Quark soft cheese
2 tbsp artificial sweetener
2–3 drops vanilla essence
2 amaretti biscuits, crushed
2 tsp Amaretto (Italian almond liqueur), optional

To decorate
chopped mint leaves

1. Cut the nectarines in half and remove the stones.

2. In a bowl, mix together the Quark, sweetener, vanilla, amaretti biscuits and Amaretto, if using.

3. Place three nectarine halves, cut side up, on each serving plate and carefully spoon the amaretti mixture into the centre of each nectarine half. Decorate with mint leaves and serve immediately.

raspberry and custard
frozen mousse

A quick-and-easy dessert, ideal for a hot summer's day. Just make sure you've got plenty in the freezer.

SERVES 4 Ⓥ ❄

Syns per serving
Original: 7
Green: 7

Preparation time 15 minutes
plus freezing

600g/1lb 6oz raspberries
4–5 tbsp artificial sweetener
500g/1lb 2oz low fat Devon custard
200g/7oz very low fat natural fromage frais

To decorate
berries

1. Place the raspberries and sweetener in a food processor and blend for a few seconds until roughly puréed.

2. Place the custard in a shallow, freezerproof container and stir through the fromage frais and the raspberry mixture. Place in the freezer for 2–3 hours and then lightly beat with a fork, every 30–40 minutes for the next few hours to break up the ice crystals, until the mousse has firmed up and is set. Alternatively, if you have an ice-cream maker, put the mixture in the container and proceed according to the manufacturer's instructions.

3. To serve the mousse, place 1–2 scoops on chilled serving plates and decorate with berries.

blackberry and filo stacks

This is an impressive-looking dessert that needs eating quickly to enjoy at its best (this won't be a problem). Assemble it at the last minute if you can.

MAKES 4 Ⓥ

Syns per serving
Original: 4½
Green: 4½

Preparation time 15 minutes
Cooking time about 14 minutes

4 x 25g/1oz sheets of filo pastry
8 tbsp very low fat natural fromage frais
1 tbsp artificial sweetener
1 tsp finely grated lemon zest
200g/7oz blackberries

To decorate
½ tsp icing sugar

1. Preheat the oven to 200°C/Gas 6. Prepare a large baking sheet by lining it with baking parchment. Cut each filo sheet into nine 7.5cm/3in squares and place on the prepared baking sheet. Place another sheet of parchment over the filo and place another baking sheet on top.

2. Bake in the oven for 8 minutes and then remove the top baking sheet and parchment and return the filo squares to the oven for another 5–6 minutes, to crisp up. Remove and allow to cool. Set aside.

3. Meanwhile, whisk together the fromage frais, sweetener and lemon zest.

4. To assemble the dessert, place three filo squares on a serving plate and spoon over 2 tbsp of the fromage frais mixture. Top with half the fruit and top yet again with three more filo squares. Repeat with the fromage frais mixture and fruit, ending with the remaining filo squares. Dust lightly with icing sugar and serve.

kiwi, pineapple and orange sundaes

**The unanimous verdict on this really simple, juicy, fruity dessert will be,
'Please Mum, can we have some more?'**

SERVES 4 ⓥ

Syns per serving
Original: 4
Green: 4

Preparation time 10 minutes

8 large kiwi fruit, peeled and sliced

400g/14oz fresh pineapple, cut into bite-sized pieces

400g/14oz orange segments

500g/1lb 2oz very low fat pineapple or tropical flavoured yogurt

4 x 50g/2oz scoops of reduced fat soft-scoop ice cream

1. Place four large sundae glasses on a work surface and layer each one with the kiwi fruit, pineapple, orange and yogurt.

2. Top each serving with a scoop of ice cream and serve immediately.

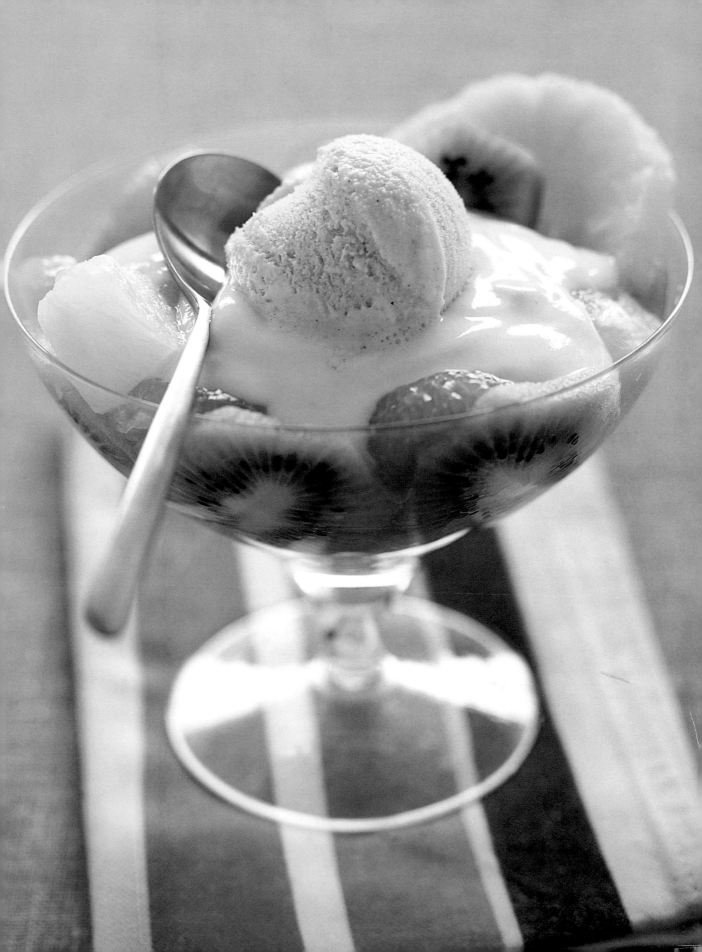

passionfruit and mango eton mess

At last, a meringue dessert that doesn't need a meringue that's in perfect condition. Hooray for Eton!

SERVES 4 Ⓥ

Syns per serving
Original: 3
Green: 3

Preparation time 10 minutes

2 large mangoes
4 meringue nests
400g/14oz Müllerlight vanilla yogurt
2 drops vanilla essence
2 tsp finely grated orange zest
pulp and seeds of
4 passionfruit

To decorate
mango slices

1. Peel, stone and finely chop the mango flesh, reserving some slices for decoration.

2. Over a large bowl, lightly crush the meringue nests with your hands into small pieces.

3. Place the yogurt in a separate bowl and stir in the vanilla essence, orange zest and passionfruit pulp and seeds.

4. Layer the chopped mango, yogurt mixture and crushed meringue in four chilled dessert bowls. Decorate with mango slices and serve immediately.

cinnamon poached pears

These pears are poached with cinnamon and topped with creamy fromage frais. Desserts don't come much easier than this.

SERVES 4 Ⓥ

Syns per serving
Original: 3½
Green: 3½

Preparation time 10 minutes
Cooking time 10–12 minutes

250ml/9fl oz diluted sugar-free Ribena

2 sticks of cinnamon

2 cloves

1 tsp ground cinnamon

2 tbsp golden caster sugar

1–2 tbsp artificial sweetener

450g/1lb pears, peeled, halved and cored

To serve

very low fat natural fromage frais

1. Pour the diluted Ribena into a saucepan and add the cinnamon sticks, cloves, ground cinnamon, sugar, sweetener and pears. Place over a medium heat and bring to the boil. Cover, reduce the heat and simmer gently for 6–8 minutes or until the pears are just tender. Remove the pears with a slotted spoon and transfer to a serving dish.

2. Bring the syrup in the pan to the boil and remove from the heat. Strain into a jug and pour over the pears.

3. To serve, place the pears and the warm syrup in bowls and serve with spoonfuls of the fromage frais.

choco espresso cups

This 'mousse' has orange zest added, which contrasts beautifully with the rich coffee taste. The only problem is that one is never enough.

SERVES 4 Ⓥ

Syns per serving
Original: 1½
Green: 1½

Preparation time 10 minutes
plus chilling

1 tsp strong instant espresso coffee dissolved in 2 tsp water

125g/4½oz very low fat natural fromage frais

125g/4½oz Quark soft cheese

1 tsp finely grated orange zest

1 tbsp granulated artificial sweetener

1 tsp vanilla essence

2 tsp drinking chocolate

To serve

very low fat natural fromage frais

1 tsp chocolate vermicelli

8 chocolate covered coffee beans

1. In a large bowl, whisk together the coffee, fromage frais, Quark, orange zest, sweetener, vanilla essence and drinking chocolate until creamy.

2. Divide the mixture between four cappuccino cups or dessert tumblers and place in the fridge until they have firmed up and are well chilled.

3. Before serving, top with a teaspoonful of fromage frais, sprinkle with the chocolate vermicelli and finish with a couple of coffee beans. Serve immediately.

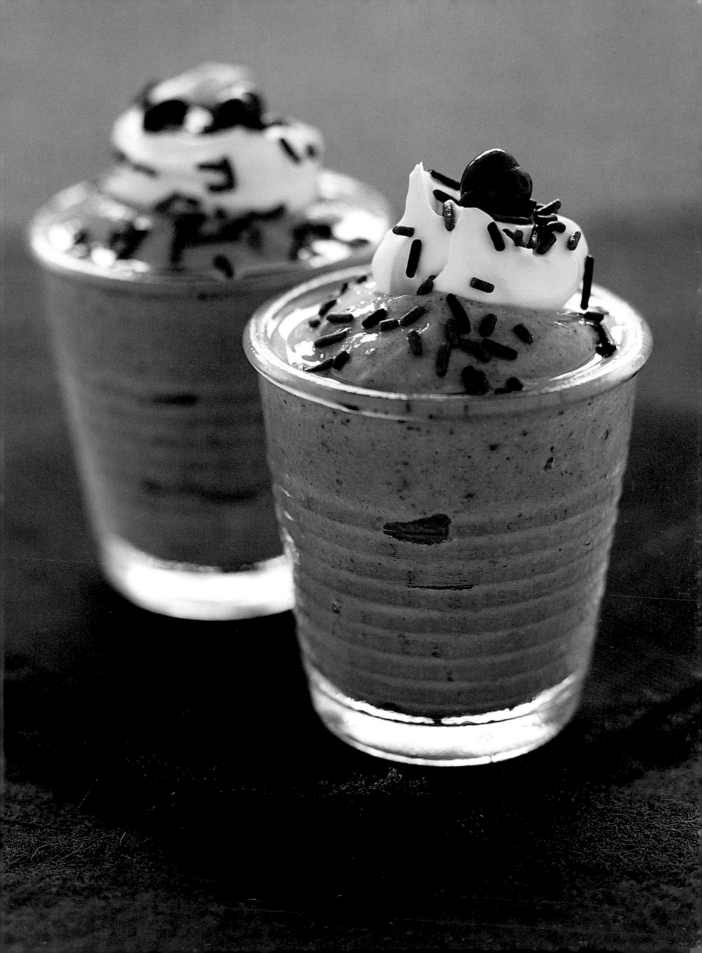

fruity yogurt
ice lollies

These fruity yogurt ice lollies not only save on Syns, they also save you pounds on the ice-cream van variety.

MAKES 4 Ⓥ ❄

Syns per serving
Original: Free
Green: Free

Preparation time 5 minutes plus freezing

250g/9oz Müllerlight vanilla yogurt

350g/12oz diced mixed fruit of your choice (e.g. apricots, plums, peaches, pineapple)

1 tsp artificial sweetener

1–2 drops vanilla extract

1. In a bowl, mix the yogurt with the fruit, sweetener and vanilla extract. Carefully spoon the mixture into four ice-lolly moulds, insert an ice-cream stick in the centre of each one and then freeze for 4–6 hours until firm.

2. To serve, dip the moulds in hot water for a few seconds and remove carefully. Serve immediately.

strawberry ripple cups

Home-grown strawberries mixed with strawberry yogurt, smothered in natural yogurt and topped with crushed biscuits make a wonderful summer dessert.

SERVES 4 ⓥ ❋ (yogurt and fruit only)

Syns per serving
Original: 2½
Green: 2½

Preparation time 10 minutes

800g/1lb 12oz strawberries

400g/14oz Müllerlight strawberry yogurt

200g/7oz very low fat natural yogurt

3 amaretti biscuits, roughly crushed

To serve

a small dollop of very low fat natural yogurt

chopped mint leaves

strawberries

1. Place 400g/14oz of the strawberries in a food processor and blend until smooth. Set aside.

2. In a large mixing bowl, add the strawberry yogurt and the remaining strawberries. Mix together.

3. Place a spoonful of the strawberry yogurt mixture into the base of four chilled dessert glasses. Divide the natural yogurt on top and spoon over the strawberry purée. Sprinkle over the crushed biscuits and top each serving with a small dollop of yogurt, mint leaves and strawberries. Serve immediately.

iced strawberry hearts

Strawberries and 'cream' – with a difference! Show them how much you care with this heart-healthy version. Wouldn't this make a lovely Valentine's Day dessert?

MAKES 4 Ⓥ ❄

Syns per serving
Original: 1½
Green: 1½

Preparation time
5 minutes plus freezing

300g/11oz fresh or good quality frozen strawberries, hulled and roughly chopped

4 tsp artificial sweetener

300g/11oz Müllerlight strawberry yogurt

1. Place the strawberries and 2 teaspoons sweetener in a food processor and blend until smooth.

2. Fill four individual heart moulds halfway up with the strawberry purée and freeze for several hours or until set.

3. Stir the remaining sweetener into the yogurt and pour over the strawberry purée. Place back in the freezer until completely frozen.

4. Dip the moulds in hot water for a few seconds to release and pop them in the fridge for 5–10 minutes before serving.

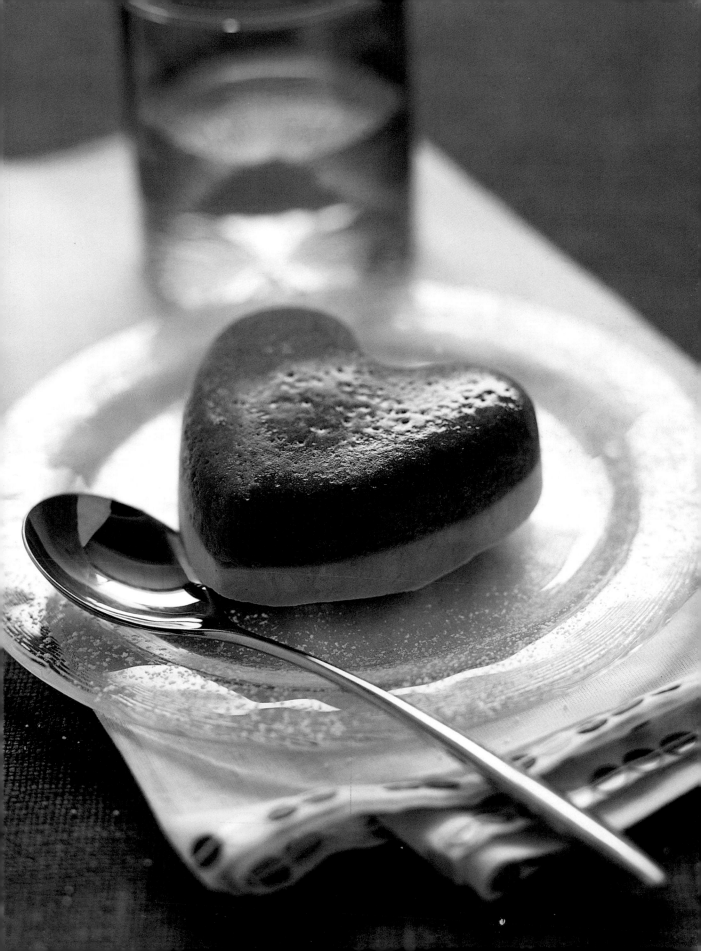

food
optimising
a powerfully liberating weight-loss system

Slimming World, the UK's leading slimming organisation, has been helping people reshape their lives for almost four decades. Launched in 1969 by founder Margaret Miles-Bramwell, the company continually pushes the boundaries with its pioneering approach to weight management.

It is a testament to the success of that unique approach that, while keeping pace with the latest nutrition guidelines and changing lifestyles, the basic principles have stayed constant. Food Optimising, the eating plan at the heart of those principles, turns the old-fashioned idea about diets and deprivation on its head. This is a liberating weight-loss system like no other because it:

- **Banishes hunger:** you can pile your plate high with delicious, satisfying food, every meal, every day. And still lose weight beautifully.
- **Frees you to eat:** no foods are banned. You're in control and YOU make the choice about what, where and when to eat. At last you can relax around food and enjoy it, including your favourite treats!
- **Offers you choice:** no other eating plan is more liberal, more flexible, more friendly.
- **Lets you be wonderfully human:** you never need to feel guilty again. You never need to start all over again. You can understand and control your behaviour around food.

- **Really takes care of you:** relish the food you eat, safe in the knowledge that all your nutritional needs are being met.

How many people say 'diet' and mean deprivation? It doesn't have to be that way – in fact, experts agree too-strict diets can actually slow down your weight loss. If it's too restrictive, you risk losing lean tissue as well as body fat, and that can slow down your metabolic rate. And so many 'diets' fail because they leave you craving your favourite foods – only a superhuman could keep it up and maintain weight losses over a very long period.

To lose weight and keep it off, it's important to make healthy eating choices a part of everyday life. Experts recommend gradual weight loss based on a sensible ceiling on calories. Food Optimising follows this tenet but in a way that's so clever and freeing that you never even have to think about counting the calories or running out of options.

Food Optimising has been called sophistication made simple. That's because it's rather like a set of traffic lights in the rush hour. It gives you the GREEN light to eat limitless amounts from a long list of deliciously satisfying healthy foods, which we call Free Foods. Then it shines the AMBER light on certain foods that are needed in measured amounts to ensure you're getting a good

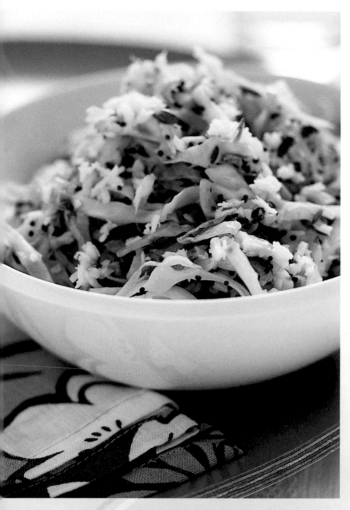
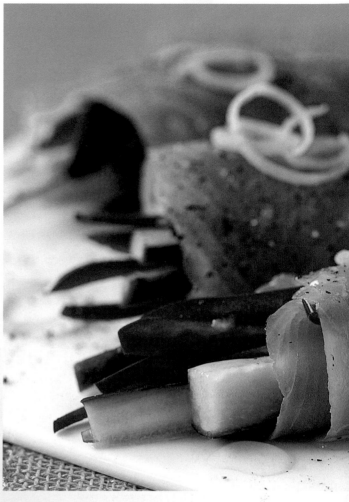

nutritional balance – we call these Healthy Extras. Food Optimising also flags up the RED light on other foods that we can enjoy in more controlled amounts.

GREEN LIGHT FOR FREE FOODS

This is the foundation on which Food Optimising is based. These are foods that you can eat in unlimited amounts – any time, anywhere! Food Optimising gives you the choice of hundreds of delicious, satisfying everyday foods that you can eat freely – with NO limits, no measuring, no weighing and no counting. Fill up on these Free Foods and you need never go hungry. These are wholesome, everyday foods that are relatively low in calories but high in hunger satisfaction –

so you don't feel the need to fill up so often.

You're encouraged to fill up on Free Foods as much as you need to satisfy your appetite. Healthy eating guidelines recommend at least five servings of fruit and vegetables a day but with most of them Free Foods, you can enjoy as many as you like.

AMBER LIGHT FOR HEALTHY EXTRAS

Each day you are asked to choose three or four times from a long list of choices that will give your body the vital vitamins, minerals and fibre it needs. Healthy Extras include milk and cheese for calcium, and wholemeal bread and breakfast cereals for fibre.

- **The Original choice:** if your idea of heaven is roast beef, fish and seafood and traditional cooked breakfasts, this is the choice for you. This plan allows unlimited lean beef, lamb, pork, chicken, turkey, fish and seafood plus fresh fruit and most vegetables, very low fat natural yogurt and fromage frais.

- **The Green choice:** ideal for those who are happy to eat less meat and love to fill up on pasta, jacket potatoes, vegetable curries, rice, baked beans, pulses and grains. Perfect for vegetarians and vegans, it also sets no limits on vegetables, fresh fruit, very low fat natural yogurt and fromage frais.

Some foods are Free whatever option you take – these are known as Superfree Foods. They include most vegetables and fruits, and some dairy products, including Quark and very low fat natural cottage cheese.

- **Mix2Max:** maximise your freedom with the option to switch plans throughout the day. Mix2Max lets you make your choice one meal at a time, so you can go Original for breakfast, Green for lunch and back to Original for supper if the fancy takes you.

- **Success Express:** is designed to give your weight loss a boost without leaving you hungry. It also allows you free rein to eat Green and Original Free Foods together in one meal.

- **Free2Go:** Slimming World was the first slimming organisation to offer free support to young people with weight concerns. Free2Go was devised with their needs in mind and is a specially 'liberated' plan that helps them to make healthy eating a lifelong habit. Find out more on page 210.

RED LIGHT FOR SYNS

And still there's more to enjoy! Syns – short for 'synergy' (the way the elements of Food Optimising add up to provide an even more powerful answer to the misery weight problems can bring) allow you to carry on enjoying your favourite treats. You're free to enjoy chocolate, cake, crisps and alcohol. Simply count its unique Syn value and enjoy your daily Syn allowance, which will depend on your weight, height and lifestyle.

Three simple steps to the great health highway … and still there are more routes to choose from! Slimming World has developed a number of choices to ensure that anyone, whatever their tastes and lifestyle, can realise their dream. Just look at the choices in the box above.

As with any weight-loss programme, Food Optimising requires some changes to the way you shop, cook and eat. The great news is that these are easy, realistic changes that not only bring health benefits but which can also amaze you with the results.

And because Food Optimising is so liberal and enjoyable, it's easy to adopt as a habit for life. A liberating, wonderful life.

image therapy

light years ahead

As if the everyday ups and downs of life are not enough, we live in a world driven to be 'celebrity-slim' among a population that has never been so overweight. The unwritten rules of society say that, to be beautiful and admired, to be 'worthy' of praise, we have to be a certain shape, a certain size – both small! The larger we get, it seems, the more invisible we become. We really like to be tough on ourselves, don't we?

Is there any wonder we sometimes feel obliged to beat ourselves up for having the audacity to be imperfect? We view ourselves as failures, as worthless. If we've tried and failed to slim alone, it's so hard to stay focused and motivated, especially with such a poor view of our chance of ultimate success.

Slimming World's unique brand of support recognises and addresses these problems – that's the reason our groups are such a powerhouse of inspiration, motivation and success. At its very heart is Image Therapy, a support system based on group participation that's light years ahead of others. It invites people to feel good about themselves, to forgive themselves for past failures and to know that their dreams can be realised.

But Image Therapy never loses touch with reality. Rather, it raises a member's awareness that they are at the controls when it comes to shaping the future.

BALANCING ACT

It's as well to remember that excess weight doesn't automatically result from gluttony. Overeating simply means taking in more calories than we expend. That doesn't have to mean excessive eating, it might reflect a small but gradual increase in our intake of calorie-rich foods. It can also happen if our activity levels fall slightly as we get older. Quite small changes can add up to extra weight gain.

Losing it again is one of the hardest challenges we might ever deal with. People who have never had to struggle with weight, never faced the pain of failing, often cannot comprehend the emotional and psychological upheaval and distress that results. Overcoming what might be a lifetime habit alone can be an enormous, uphill struggle, so often doomed to fail at the first hurdle.

Image Therapy is like a warm blanket that wraps itself around you. IMAGE stands for Individual Motivation and Group Experience. Everyone in a group can tap into the shared experiences, power, love and support of their fellow members.

It really is a voyage of self-discovery that makes the slimming experience truly exciting, because anything is possible with the support of like-minded people, which is exactly what you'll find at a Slimming World group.

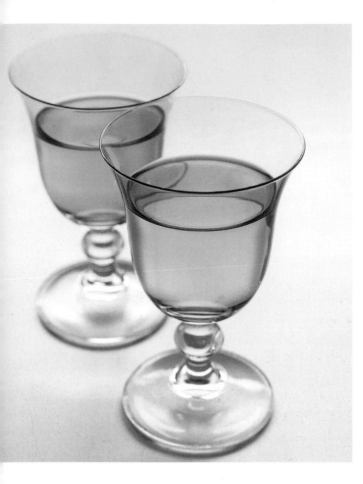

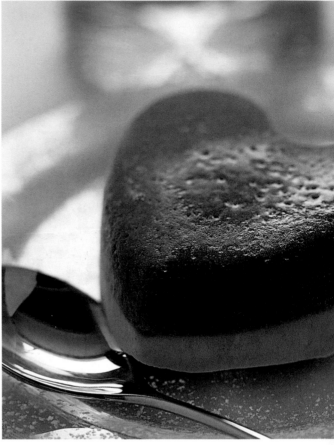

MUTUAL SUPPORT

Your Consultant is someone who knows from experience exactly what it is like to have a weight problem – because they've been there too. It really matters to them that you get where you want to be and they will be with you every step of the way. And as well as the benefit of your Consultant's experience, you have the pooled resources, suggestions, support, experiences and triumphs of your fellow group members to help keep you motoring.

Group Therapy has long been recognised as a powerful way of supporting people as they go through changes in their life. It's particularly effective when the group shares a common goal. Team spirit and laughter are both to the fore and a kind of magic begins to emerge. The more you share thoughts and ideas with others, the stronger your own motivation becomes.

In practical terms, Image Therapy helps by breaking down the psychological barriers that so often lead slimmers to feel demoralised and worthless – and that's just a small step from giving up.

At Slimming World, we believe that if you make a mistake, slip a little or have a bad week, it's a sign you're human, not that you're a failure! It's no crime. You don't need forgiveness. In fact, if you have put on weight between meetings, you're more likely to get a pat on the back than admonishment – why? Because we have all been there and how much easier would it have been to stay at home than face the scales that week?

Even if you arrived feeling a little less than inspired, you can leave feeling motivated and supported, ready to get right back on the road to success.

body
magic
an active interest in your health

Most of us don't need to be told that losing weight is about using up more calories than we take in, we just need understanding and support to help us do it. That's what Food Optimising and Image Therapy is all about.

And so it is with the dreaded 'E' word ... exercise! Of course, no one likes to be told time and again that if we want to be fit and healthy and keep our 'bits' in good working order into old age, we need to get out there and moving! If only it was that easy. Well, that's what Body Magic is all about.

Body Magic is a programme, unique to Slimming World, which offers extra rewards for members who build regular activity into their routine. Members are encouraged to start at a realistic level and work at their own pace, building up gradually until Body Magic becomes a lifelong habit.

We know trainers and tracksuits don't appeal to everyone, and there's never any question of pushing members into aerobics classes and trendy gym membership. Indeed, it's possible to pursue your weight-loss dream through diet alone without doing any exercise at all.

While it's reasonable to expect to lose 1–2lbs each week through Food Optimising alone, moderate activity can boost that weight loss and bring all kinds of health benefits – it can even help to lengthen your life!

START SLOWLY

Body Magic isn't about push-ups or pounding the streets. It's a way of bringing moderate activity into your daily routine and making it a lifetime habit. It reflects extensive research that points to the fact that the best way to lose weight – and to keep it off long term – is by combining regular moderate activity with a healthy eating plan.

Every step counts as members are encouraged to begin gently, building to 10 minutes a day for five days of the week, increasing to blocks of 15 minutes six times a week and with the long-term goal of 30 minutes a day for five days of the week. Milestones are celebrated through a series of Body Magic awards – bronze, silver, gold and platinum.

Numerous studies confirm that building some kind of regular activity into our normal routine is one of the best ways to keep weight off. And when you consider that most of us put on weight because our activity levels have dropped, that really does make sense.

If you compare your lifestyle with that of your grandparents, the difference in activity levels soon becomes clear. Thirty years ago people were generally a third more active than we are today. When you consider that most families have at least one car in daily use, walking and cycling to school is less common and outdoor play is now less popular than computer games and television, *yet we still eat, on average, the same amount*, there's little wonder that our sedentary lifestyle is reflected on the scales.

The good news is that relatively small changes can make a big difference in terms of boosting weight loss and improving our overall health prospects. Health experts agree that just three or four sessions of moderate activity a week can boost weight loss by 1–2lbs a month. That might not sound dramatic – and yet it adds up to 12–24lbs a year! There is also a host of other benefits to be gained from making moderate exercise a regular routine (see the box, below).

The benefits of moderate, regular exercise

- You will tone and firm your muscles, increase calorie-consumption and boost the amount of fat you lose.
- Increasing your muscle:fat ratio increases your metabolism, so you're more likely to keep the weight off.
- Activity suppresses appetite – you're less likely to overeat afterwards.
- Activity helps to lower blood pressure and reduce the risk of heart disease.
- It can strengthen muscles and build stronger bones and joints.
- It's a great stress relief and a wonderful mood booster. You're less inclined to turn to food for comfort.
- Energy levels climb, both physically and mentally.
- Self-confidence soars as you make positive changes to your lifestyle.

WATCH THE RESULTS

Slimming World has created Body Magic as a way of translating all this fantastic news into practical, achievable results. You don't have to do masses of activity to feel the benefits – research shows that the heavier you are, the more benefit you get out of any activity you do. Just putting a little 'oomph' into the housework, getting out and walking the dog, cycling, shopping, gardening and dancing can all help you build more success – and enjoyment – into your weight-loss journey.

Choosing an activity you enjoy or inviting a friend or family member to join you are good incentives for keeping up the momentum. So you could start off, for example, with a five-minute walk and then aim to continue this every day for a week. The following week build to seven or ten minutes a day, so you can gauge your progress. You'll soon start feeling the benefits. And it's never too late to start.

Slimming World members are always happy to suggest ways of getting into an active routine, such as taking a short walk at work before sitting down to your lunchtime sandwich, cancelling your newspaper delivery order and walking to pick up a copy from the newsagent or riding your bike to and from work.

And it's just as vital you don't try to tackle too much too soon. You are less likely to succeed in the long term if you get too serious about an exercise routine, worry about missing the odd session or adopt an all-or-nothing approach. It's far better to build a regular routine that you know you will be able to make a permanent feature of your normal lifestyle. You can't store up the good you're doing yourself from activity – the key to making it work is to keep it going!

family
health
on a plate!

Health and parenting experts, child psychologists and even the government agree that getting families back together around the table at mealtimes is one of the most positive things we can do for our children. In a TV and internet-dominated world of chilled dinners and meals on trays, not only can family meals based on fresh ingredients save preparation time – and money – it's a wonderful chance to relax together, strengthen family bonds and help our children build social skills.

It's also a marvellous opportunity to ensure we share a nutritious, balanced and varied diet, which can make a difference to the whole family's long-term health prospects. The tempting family recipes in this book will show how mouth-watering menus and healthy eating go together deliciously. No one ever needs to miss out on their favourite foods and everyone is free to enjoy family meals.

Slimming World feels a duty to share the insight and expertise amassed over more than three-and-a-half decades of conquering the practical and social problems so many people encounter around food. When our organisation was launched, obesity was, by and large, a 'grown-ups' problem. Today, our younger generation stand on the front line of what has been labelled a health 'time bomb'.

We saw childhood obesity in the UK rise alarmingly from 9.6 per cent in 1995 to 13.7 per

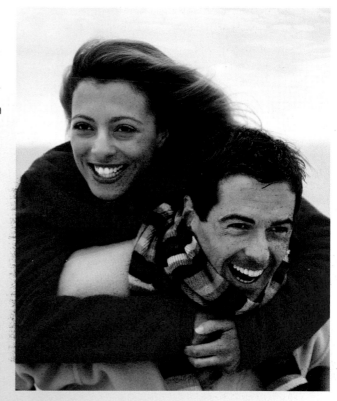

cent in 2003. Indeed, research among Slimming World's 250,000 members suggests that a fifth of parents are worried about the weight of one or more of their children. We realise that our children's futures rely heavily on the values and habits they learn at home. Our research also shows how parents can have a powerful, positive influence on children's eating choices – a *Slimming World Magazine* survey revealed that three-quarters of people who use Food

Optimising – members and non-members alike – feel they influence other family members to eat more healthily. Encouraged by this feedback, we felt compelled to act.

IT'S A FAMILY AFFAIR

So in January 2006 we became the first and only national organisation to offer free advice and support to young people aged 11 to 15 who have weight concerns – through the launch of Family Affair, an initiative that helps make it easier for everyone to address the issue of healthy eating together as a family.

Slimming World is well equipped to help address the rise in obesity. Not only do we have an understanding, built over decades, of what causes us to become and stay overweight and how to counter it, our unique system goes much further. That's because we have a much deeper understanding of the psychological factors that so often stop individuals conquering their weight problems. A Slimming World member is never judged, preached to or told what to weigh or what they should look like. We put all the choices in members' hands and they have responded in their thousands – by changing their lives.

Since its launch, thousands of families have signed up for the Family Affair scheme. The company, through its network of 5,500 groups, provides them with the combination of professional help, a warm, supportive environment and practical solutions that have proved difficult to find elsewhere.

Family Affair provides real support for families and offers extra benefits for groups, children, senior citizens and students. The scheme allows up to four members of a family to attend group meetings together for a specially discounted joining and group fee. Students and senior citizens can claim discounts for regular attendance and, for the first time, meetings were opened up to 11 to 15 year olds who can attend free of charge, with medical consent, when accompanied by a fee-paying parent or guardian.

There is no pressure to lose weight – no youngster need ever step on the scales if they don't wish to. The focus is always on health and on achievable levels of activity. Children and young people are always encouraged to make their own healthy eating choices and enjoy a wide range of foods. This is done through Free2Go, a 'super-liberated' weight-management system based on Food Optimising. Perfect for mums-to-be as well as growing children who want to 'grow into' their weight or simply eat more healthily, the plan offers so much freedom.

Our ultimate aim is to help children to eat more of the healthy and satisfying foods that fill us up for longer, and to cut down on foods that are high in fat and sugar.

Just as important is the warmth and encouragement they receive in Group. There they have the support of their parent or guardian and their dedicated Slimming World Consultant and fellow members.

Free2Go

With Free2Go, you can:

- Fill up on unlimited Free Foods, with no weighing or calorie counting.
- Mix Green and Original Free Foods freely.
- Enjoy unlimited Healthy Extras, with certain small exceptions.
- Have more freedom with Syns, aiming instead to make 'cool swaps' as often as possible with Free Food or Healthy Extra choices – for example, switching from sugar-coated cereal to porridge or Weetabix – and ultimately to limit Syn choices to one a day.

30-minute meal
menus

Take a week or two to follow our tasty selection of mouth-watering menus and you'll be able to plan your shopping with confidence. You'll soon discover that not only does Food Optimising work, it's fabulously simple too!

These menus are designed to help you understand the variety of meals that are possible when you start Food Optimising (we've included lots of meals that the whole family will enjoy!). You can be sure of plenty of nourishing, satisfying food that will keep you full and healthy – and help you lose weight too! We've included some of the recipes featured in this book.

Here's how to use Food Optimising menus most effectively:

1. Decide whether you wish to have a Green or Original day and stick to that choice all day. You can make every day a Green day or include some Original days too. Within the Green menus we have included meat-free choices suitable for vegetarians.
2. Pick one breakfast, one lunch and one dinner from your chosen set.
3. Choose around 10–15 Syns-worth of food from the Syns list on page 220. Some Food Optimisers find they lose weight best on 5 Syns, others on 20 Syns. On some days, you might find you perhaps need to use 30, if you are going out or celebrating. In general, we

find 10 Syns a day is a good rule of thumb for effective weight loss.
4. Each day, choose twice from the following milk and cheese lists to boost your calcium intake, which is vital for a healthy diet.

MILK
350ml/12fl oz skimmed milk/unsweetened calcium-enriched soya milk
225ml/8fl oz semi-skimmed milk
175ml/6fl oz whole milk
225ml/8fl oz sweetened calcium-enriched soya milk

CHEESE
25g/1oz Cheddar
25g/1oz Edam
25g/1oz Gouda
40g/1½oz mozzarella
40g/1½oz reduced fat Cheddar/Cheshire
3 Dairylea Original triangles
2 mini Babybel cheeses

On the menus given on the following pages – divided into Green days and Original days – check out the foods marked in bold. These can be eaten freely without any weighing or measuring. Fill up on these foods when you feel peckish. You can also turn to our Free Food list on pages 218–19 and select other Free Foods to enjoy whenever you want, in whatever quantity you want.

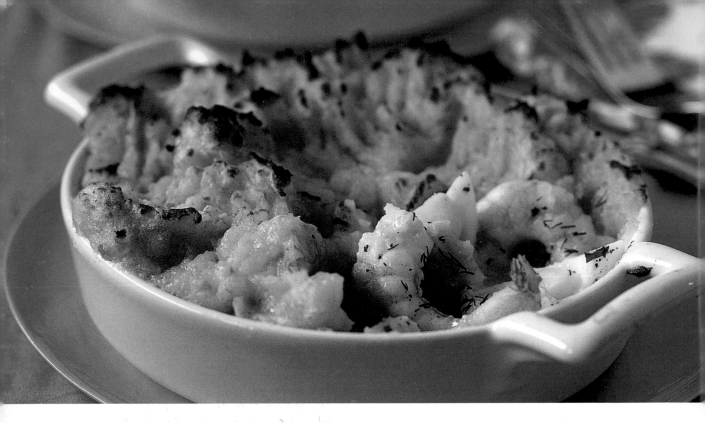

- Eating at least two portions of fish a week, of which one is an oily fish.
- Aiming to keep your salt intake to no more than 6g a day (1 level teaspoon). As well as limiting the amount of table salt you add to food, watch out for salt added to manufactured foods and sauces. Try flavouring foods with herbs and spices instead.
- Remembering the latest recommendations regarding intake of fluids, which is to aim for six to eight cups, mugs or glasses of any type of fluid per day (excluding alcohol).

Maximise your healthy eating by:
- Eating at least five portions of fresh fruit and vegetables every day. Frozen fruit and frozen and canned vegetables can also be used.
- Trimming any visible fat off meat and removing any skin from poultry.
- Varying your choices as much as possible to ensure you have the widest range of nutrients in your diet.

Note for Slimming World members: Healthy Extra B choices are built into the menus.

When you have experienced the pleasure of Food Optimising on your plate you will want to design your own menus. You can do this with the complete Food Optimising system, available at Slimming World groups throughout the UK.

green menus

MENUS 213

BREAKFASTS

1. Fresh **melon wedges** followed by 25g/1oz Nestlé Honey Nut Shredded Wheat served with milk from the allowance and topped with lots of fresh **strawberries**.

2. Two slices of wholemeal toast smothered in **spaghetti hoops** or **baked beans in tomato sauce** followed by an **apple** and a **banana**.

3. Fresh **grapefruit** followed by 40g/1½oz Nestlé Fibre 1 served with milk from the allowance and a pot of **Nestlé Sveltesse 0% Fat Yogurt**.

4. A large fluffy **omelette** filled with 25g/1oz grated Cheddar cheese and served with plenty of grilled **mushrooms** and **tomatoes** and **baked beans in tomato sauce** followed by **fresh fruit** of your choice.

5. Layer a pot of **Müllerlight Yogurt** with 25g/1oz Kellogg's Fruit 'n' Fibre and lots of fresh or frozen **berries** in a tall glass.

6. Boiled **eggs** served with 'soldiers' cut from two slices of wholemeal toast and spread with Marmite followed by a **fresh fruit** salad smothered in **very low fat natural yogurt**.

7. Large bowl of fresh **orange** and **grapefruit segments** followed by 25g/1oz Weetabix Mini Crisp served with milk from the allowance and topped with lots of sliced **banana**.

8. **Quorn sausages**, any variety, grilled and served with lots of grilled **tomatoes** and **onion** wedges, scrambled **egg** and two slices of wholemeal toast followed by slices of fresh **pineapple**.

9. 25g/1oz Kellogg's All Bran Bran Flakes topped with lots of fresh **raspberries** and served with milk from the allowance followed by a **pear** and a **satsuma**.

10. Three rashers grilled lean bacon served with an **egg** fried in Fry Light and plenty of grilled **tomatoes** and **mushrooms** followed by a **peach** or **nectarine**.

LUNCHES

* denotes recipe suggestion with picture

1. **Ratatouille Jackets** (see page 46*) served with a large crisp **salad**. Enjoy 350g/12oz canned pears in juice topped with lashings of **very low fat natural yogurt** for afters.

2. 75g/3oz grilled lean gammon served with heaps of **potato** slices sautéed in Fry Light and lots of grilled **mushrooms** and **baked beans in tomato sauce**. Follow with **fresh fruit** of your choice.

3. **Lemon, Courgette and Minted Pea Fusilli** (see page 160*), followed by 400g/14oz fruit cocktail canned in juice and topped with **Danone Shape Lasting Satisfaction Yogurt**.

4. Two slices of wholemeal bread filled with slices of hard-boiled **egg** and juicy **tomato** and lots of baby **salad leaves**. Follow with some fresh **plums**.

5. Mix 110g/4oz tuna (in brine) with lots of cooked **pasta** shapes, chopped **cucumber**, **cherry tomatoes**, mixed **peppers** and **spring onions** and drizzle with fat-free salad dressing, plus a large bunch of **grapes**.

6. A large fluffy **omelette** filled with 75g/3oz lean diced ham served with a huge jacket **potato** and lots of grilled **tomatoes**, followed by a large bowl of **summer berries** smothered in **Müllerlight Yogurt**.

7. 110g/4oz grilled chicken breast served with **Mixed Vegetable Pad Thai** (see page 151) and a huge mixed **salad**, followed with a Kiwi, Pineapple and Orange Sundae (see page 192*).

8. Herbed Chickpea and Tabbouleh Salad (see page 55) served with a 50g/2oz crusty wholemeal roll, followed by a bowl of chopped **melon**, **kiwi** and **strawberries** smothered in **very low fat natural yogurt**.

9. 75g/3oz lean roast beef, served with plenty of mashed **potatoes** and dry-roast **potatoes** and heaps of **cabbage**, **carrots**, **peas** and **cauliflower**. Follow with a Choco Espresso Cup (see page 196*).

10. 150g/5oz cod fillet, poached or grilled, served with mountains of **Lemon Roasted Baby New Potatoes** (see page 126), **Grilled Balsamic Asparagus** (see page 134) and plenty of **baby whole sweetcorn** and **carrots**. Follow with slices of juicy fresh **pineapple**.

DINNERS

* denotes recipe suggestion with picture

1. Have a warming bowl of **Tomato, Rice and Pea Soup** (see page 16*) and follow with lots of sliced **banana** smothered in **very low fat natural yogurt** and sprinkled with nutmeg.

2. **Mexican Vegetable Rice** (see page 164*) followed by a Mango Posset (see page 178*).

3. A generous serving of **Broccoli and Garlic Pennette** (see page 156*), plus a **Peach and Raspberry Salad with Basil Cream** (see page 185) for afters.

4. A large **omelette** filled with chopped **peppers**, **red onion** and **sweetcorn** served with lots of baked **potato** wedges and loads of **salad**. Have half a **cantaloupe melon** filled with fresh or frozen **berries** for pud.

5. Lots of **Lemon Roasted Vegetable Couscous** (see page 171) followed by a serving of Passionfruit and Mango Eton Mess (see page 194).

6. A large jacket **potato** topped with a can of **mixed beans in chilli sauce** and served with a generous mixed **salad**, plus a **peach** and a **pear**.

7. **Mixed Bean and Barley Stew** (see page 172*) followed by a **fresh fruit salad** smothered in **Müllerlight Yogurt**.

8. Vegetable stir-fry: **broccoli** and **cauliflower** florets, chopped **carrots**, mixed **peppers**, **spring onions**, button **mushrooms**, **beansprouts** and **water chestnuts** stir-fried with garlic, herbs and soy sauce served on a bed of **noodles**. Follow with slices of fresh **pineapple**.

9. **Quorn sausages**, any variety, grilled and served with mountains of mashed **potatoes** and plenty of **Minted Mushy Peas** (see page 140), follow with a **Fruity Yogurt Ice Lolly** (see page 198).

10. **Mixed Mushroom and Pasta Gratin** (see page 159) served with lots of new **potatoes**, **mangetout**, **baby whole sweetcorn** and **peas**. Have **fresh fruit** of your choice for afters.

original menus

BREAKFASTS

1. Lots of grilled lean **bacon**, grilled **mushrooms** and **tomatoes**, and scrambled **egg**, served with two slices of wholemeal toast, plus a **banana**.

2. **Melon** boat filled with fresh **berries** topped with **Müllerlight Yogurt** and sprinkled with 25g/1oz Nestlé Triple Berry Shredded Wheat.

3. A bowl of fresh **orange** and **grapefruit segments**, followed by plenty of grilled **kippers**, grilled **onion** wedges and **tomatoes** and a poached **egg**.

4. A **banana** sliced lengthways sprinkled with 40g/1½oz All Bran Original and topped with lashings of **very low fat natural yogurt** flavoured with cinnamon.

5. 50g/2oz wholemeal roll filled with lots of grilled lean **bacon** and slices of **tomato**. Follow with **peaches** or **nectarines** chopped into a pot of **Danone Shape Solo Yogurt**.

6. Two Weetabix served with milk from the allowance and topped with lots of fresh **raspberries** or **strawberries**.

7. Two slices of wholemeal toast topped with lots of scrambled **egg** mixed with chopped **smoked salmon** and dill and served with lots of **mushrooms** sautéed in Fry Light.

8. Chunks of **fresh fruit** layered in a tall glass with **very low fat natural yogurt** and 25g/1oz Kellogg's Raisin Wheats.

9. Plenty of grilled lean **gammon**, grilled **tomatoes**, an **egg** fried in Fry Light and 150g/5oz baked beans in tomato sauce.

10. 25g/1oz Nestlé Shreddies served with milk from the allowance topped with lots of sliced **banana**.

LUNCHES

* denotes recipe suggestion with picture

1. **Salmon and Mixed Pepper Skewers** (see page 112) served with **Sautéed Mushrooms with Red Onion, Garlic and Parsley** (see page 136), a 225g/8oz (raw weight) jacket potato and a huge mixed **salad**. Follow with wedges of **melon**.

2. **Chilled Yogurt and Cucumber Soup** (see page 20*) served with a 50g/2oz crusty wholemeal roll, followed by a large bowl of **strawberries** smothered in **very low fat natural yogurt**.

3. Tuna and Courgette Stacks (see page 102*) served with 200g/7oz new potatoes in their skins and plenty of **sugar snap peas**, **baby whole sweetcorn** and **broccoli** florets. Enjoy Amaretti Stuffed Nectarines (see page 189) for pud.

4. Fill a 50g/2oz wholemeal roll with lots of sliced **turkey**, baby **salad leaves**, sliced **tomato** and hard-boiled **egg**. Chop plenty of **kiwi** and **grapes** into a pot of **Danone Shape Solo Yogurt** for afters.

5. Heaps of meaty Bolognese sauce made with extra lean minced **beef**, chopped **tomatoes**, **onion**, garlic, **peppers** and **mushrooms** and served with 100g/3½oz (boiled weight) wholemeal spaghetti, plus an **apple** and a **pear**.

6. Two slices of wholemeal bread filled with lots of sliced **turkey** breast, fresh **tomato** slices and **watercress**. Follow with sliced **banana** stirred into a pot of **Nestlé Sveltesse 0% Fat Yogurt**.

7. Combine lots of cooked **chicken** chunks with 200g/7oz cold sliced new potatoes in their skins and plenty of shredded **lettuce**, chopped **beetroot**, **celery** and **carrot**, pour over some **very low fat natural fromage frais** and mix well. Follow with a bowl of chopped **melon**, **pineapple** and **kiwi** smothered in **Müllerlight Yogurt**.

8. A large grilled lean **gammon** steak served with poached button **mushrooms**, an **egg** fried in Fry Light and 150g/5oz baked beans in tomato sauce. Follow with **fresh fruit**.

9. 225g/8oz (raw weight) jacket potato filled with lots of tuna in brine mixed with **very low fat natural cottage cheese** and chunks of fresh **pineapple** and served with a huge mixed **salad**. Follow with a bowl of fresh **berries**.

10. Plenty of lean roast **beef** served with 200g/7oz new potatoes in their skins and heaps of **carrots**, **cabbage**, **green beans** and Creamy Dijon Mustard Cauliflower Cheese (see page 137), follow with a Mixed Berry Jelly (see page 182*)

DINNERS
* denotes recipe suggestion with picture

1. **Pink Peppercorn and Salmon Pâté** (see page 29) followed by **Moroccan-style Lamb** (see page 78*) served with plenty of steamed **carrot** and **courgette** ribbons. Round off the meal with a Strawberry Ripple Cup (see page 199).

2. A large warming bowl of **Chicken and Tarragon Fricassee** (see page 72*) followed by Griddled Pineapple and Nectarine Skewers (see page 180).

3. A grilled juicy **salmon** steak served with **Roasted Stuffed Courgettes** (see page 132*) and a mixed **salad**, follow with a **fresh fruit salad** smothered in **Danone Shape Lasting Satisfaction Yogurt**.

4. **Melon** wedges, followed with Sweet and Sour Pork with Cabbage (see page 82) served with lots of **carrots**, **mangetout** and **baby whole sweetcorn**.

5. **Chicken and Mushroom Stir-fry** (see page 71) served with additional **Free vegetables** of your choice, followed by a bowl of chopped **strawberries**, **kiwi** and **grapes**.

6. **Haddock and Prawn Gratin** (see page 98*) served with heaps of **broccoli** and **green beans**, follow with a Berry Puff Tart (see page 186*).

7. **Rosemary and Garlic Pork with Butternut Squash Mash** (see page 84*) served with **Moroccan-style Carrots** (see page 138*). For afters, have a bowl of **strawberries** and **blueberries** topped with lashings of **very low fat natural yogurt**.

8. **Lamb and Spinach Curry** (see page 80) served with lots of steamed **cabbage** flavoured with cardamom and plenty of mashed **swede**. Follow with an Iced Strawberry Heart (see page 200*).

9. A griddled **tuna** steak, served with lots of roasted **red**, **yellow** and **orange pepper** chunks and Oven-roasted Tomatoes with Thyme (see page 144*). Follow with Floating Islands (see page 188).

10. Lots of lean roast **lamb**, topped with mint sauce and served with mountains of **butternut squash** mash, **cauliflower** and **broccoli**, plus slices of fresh **pineapple**.

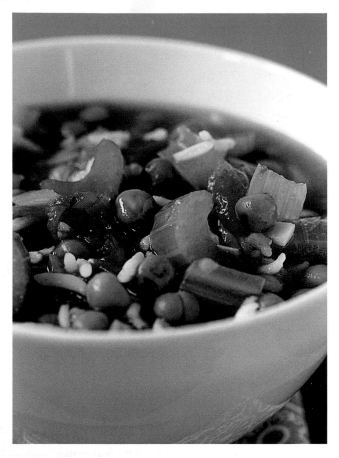
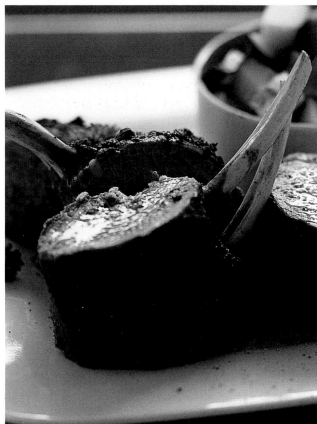
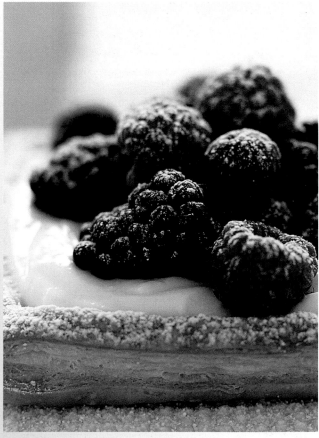
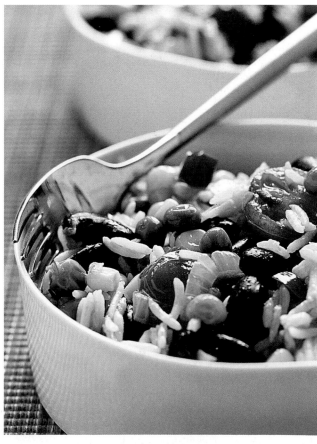

free food
selection

We have listed many of our Free Foods here. For the full list, you will need to become a Slimming World member.

KEY TO SYMBOLS

H	=	healthy
HH	=	vital to health and should be included in your diet every day
S	=	weight loss boost
SS	=	extra weight loss boost
F	=	extra fibre
FF	=	extra-rich fibre
C	=	good source of calcium
CC	=	very good source of calcium

GREEN CHOICE FREE FOODS

All vegetables are classed as a Free Food when on a Green day.

Grains, Pulses and Vegetables

Bulgur wheat	H		
Couscous	H		
Dried pasta, all types	H		
Rice, all types	H		
Baked beans	H	SS	F
Chickpeas	H		F
Lentils	H	S	F
Peas	H	SS	F
Red kidney beans	H	SS	FF
Soya beans	H		FF
Potatoes	HH		
Quorn	H	S	F
Tofu			CC

Dairy

Eggs		
Quark soft cheese	H	C
Very low fat natural cottage cheese	H	C
Very low fat natural fromage frais	H	C

Very low fat natural yogurt	H	C
Müllerlight Yogurt		C
Nestlé Sveltesse 0% Fat Yogurt		C
Shape Lasting Satisfaction Yogurt		C
Shape Solo Yogurt		C

The following fruits can be eaten freely as long as they are fresh or frozen varieties.

Fruit

Apples	HH	S
Apricots	HH	S
Bananas	HH	
Blueberries	HH	
Cherries	HH	S
Grapefruit	HH	SS
Grapes	HH	
Kiwi fruit	HH	S
Mangoes	HH	
Melon	HH	SS
Nectarines	HH	S
Oranges	HH	S
Peaches	HH	S
Pears	HH	S
Pineapple	HH	S
Plums	HH	S
Raspberries	HH	SS
Satsumas	HH	S
Strawberries	HH	SS

ORIGINAL CHOICE FREE FOODS

Not all vegetables are Free Foods on the Original Choice. Choose freely from the following list:

Vegetables

Asparagus	HH	S	
Aubergine	HH	S	
Baby whole sweetcorn	HH	S	
Beans, French/green	HH	S	
Beetroot	HH	S	
Broccoli	HH	S	
Brussels sprouts	HH		F
Cabbage	HH	S	
Carrots	HH	S	
Cauliflower	HH	S	
Celery	HH	S	
Courgettes	HH	S	
Cucumber	HH	S	
Leeks	HH	S	
Mangetout	HH	S	
Mushrooms	HH	S	
Onions	HH	S	
Peppers	HH	S	
Salad leaves	HH	S	
Spinach	HH	S	C
Spring onions	HH	S	
Squash, all types	HH	S	
Sugar snap peas	HH	S	
Swede	HH	S	
Tomatoes	HH	S	
Quorn	H	S	F
Tofu			CC

Poultry

Chicken, no fat or skin	H	S
Turkey, no fat or skin	H	S

Meat

Bacon
Beef
Gammon
Ham
Lamb
Pork

Fish

Cod	H	SS
Haddock	H	SS
Halibut	H	S
Kippers	H	
Mackerel (not smoked)	H	
Plaice	H	SS
Salmon (fresh, canned and smoked)	H	
Sole	H	SS
Tuna, canned in brine	H	S
Tuna, fresh	H	

Shellfish

Crab	H	SS	CC
Prawns	H	S	

Dairy

Eggs		
Quark soft cheese	H	C
Very low fat natural cottage cheese	H	C
Very low fat natural fromage frais	H	C
Very low fat natural yogurt	H	C
Müllerlight Yogurt		C
Nestlé Sveltesse 0% Fat Yogurt		C
Shape Lasting Satisfaction Yogurt		C
Shape Solo Yogurt		C

The following fruits can be eaten freely as long as they are fresh or frozen varieties.

Fruit

Apples	HH	S
Apricots	HH	S
Bananas	HH	
Blueberries	HH	
Cherries	HH	S
Grapefruit	HH	SS
Grapes	HH	
Kiwi fruit	HH	S
Mangoes	HH	
Melon	HH	SS
Nectarines	HH	S
Oranges	HH	S
Peaches	HH	S
Pears	HH	S
Pineapple	HH	S
Plums	HH	S
Raspberries	HH	SS
Satsumas	HH	S
Strawberries	HH	SS

syns
selection

Listed below is a selection of Syn values for foods that you can enjoy every day. You can choose 10–15 Syns each day. The values apply to both the Green and Original choices.

Alcohol	Syns
25ml/1fl oz measure of any spirit	2½
150ml/¼ pint glass of wine	5
300ml/½ pint beer/lager	5
300ml/½ pint cider	5

Biscuits, each	Syns
Cheese thin/water biscuit	1
Chocolate finger	1½
Fruit shortcake/rich tea	2
Cream cracker/cheese straw	2
Jaffa cake/ginger nut	2½
Custard cream	3
Hobnobs	3½
Chocolate digestive/Jammie Dodger	4

Cakes, each	Syns
Mr Kipling French Fancy	5½
Cadbury Mini Roll	6
Mr Kipling Country/Lemon Slice	6
Chocolate cupcake	6½
Mr Kipling Mini Battenberg	7
Individual fruit pie	9½

Chocolates and sweets, standard bag/tube, etc.	Syns
Milky Bar	3½
Fun-size bars	5
2 finger Kit Kat	5½
Fudge/Milky Way	6
Jellytots/Polo Fruits/Polo Mints	7½
Fruit Gums	8
Flake/Maltesers	9
Fruit Pastilles	10

Crisps, standard bag	Syns
French Fries/Golden Lights	4½
Quavers/Ryvita Minis	5
Seasons Crispbread Snacks	6
Snack-a-Jacks Butter Toffee Popcorn	7½
Mini Cheddars, Original	9
Walkers Crisps	9

Desserts, per pot	Syns
Müllerlight Yogurt with Cake Pieces	1
Rowntree's Ready to Eat Jelly Pot	5
Cadbury Light Chocolate Mousse (100g pot)	5½
Müllerice, Only 1% Fat	6
Danone Goodies Trifle	7½
Onken Lite Mousse	8

Ice creams/Lollies	Syns
Fruit Pastil Ice Lolly/Mini Calippo	3
50g/2oz scoop low fat ice cream	4
Fab Ice Lolly	4
Skinny Cow Iced Mini Pots	4½
Solero	5
Skinny Cow Ice Cream Cone	6
Carte D'Or Vanilla Ice Cream Tub	8½
Strawberry Cornetto	9½

Meal accompaniments, sauces and spreads	Syns
Aerosol cream: 2 level tbsp	½
Jam/marmalade: 1 level tsp	½
Mustard: 1 level tsp	½
Brown sauce/tomato ketchup: 1 level tbsp	1
Custard made with skimmed milk: 2 level tbsp	1
Gravy made without fat: 4 level tbsp	1
Honey, all varieties: 1 level tsp	1
Horseradish sauce: 1 level tbsp	1
Reduced calorie salad cream: 1 level tbsp	1½
Reduced calorie mayonnaise: 1 level tbsp	2½
Margarine/spread, low fat variety: 25g/1oz	5½
Oil, any variety: 1 level tbsp	6

index